PRAISE FOR STILL HURTING? FIND HEALTH!

"Still Hurting? FIND HEALTH! is a remarkable book. *Remarkable* is defined in Webster's as *worthy of being or likely to be noticed, especially as being uncommon or extraordinary.* This is not hyperbole but is an apt description of this monumental book. It will and should receive widespread reading and acclaim.

Although primarily directed at all people who hurt (which at one time or another is all of us), this book is an encyclopedia of the scientific and medical literature that explains how a human being is not a mind and a separated body. Human beings are highly integrated and connected systems made up of our senses, our nervous systems, our emotions, our stresses, our physiology, and our deep human spirit. As the authors say,

Disease is dysfunction, and symptoms are the expression.

Step by step, the mind-body false dichotomy is put to rest. In its place the authors carefully guide us to be fully functional and integrated human beings."

—**Clifton K. Meador, M.D.,** Executive Director Meharry-Vanderbilt Alliance
Professor of Medicine, Vanderbilt School of Medicine and Meharry Medical College
Author of *Puzzling Symptoms* and *Symptoms of Unknown Origin*

"This important book courageously details the origin of suffering for countless individuals with medically unexplained symptoms. The authors' multi-disciplined approach is learned and compassionate. They provide invaluable suggestions for a balanced physical, emotional, and spiritual life. Both text and references are superbly detailed."

—**Paul Dusseau, M.D.,** Family Physician, Columbus, Ohio

"As a psychologist in private practice, I see many patients in unexplained pain and distress. This book provides a needed resource to help others feel understood, empowered, and hopeful as they learn how the body and mind are connected. It is helpful to have a resource that covers so many topics on medically unexplained symptoms, yet it is easy to read and comprehend. The authors guide the reader from the beginning of their frustrating journey of pain to a place of encouragement with such sensitivity. I feel confident recommending *Still Hurting? FIND HEALTH!* as a resource to patients, colleagues and friends."

—**Shannon H. Johnson, Psy.D.,** Clinical Psychologist, Columbus, Ohio

"*Still Hurting? FIND HEALTH!* by Dr. William Salt II and the Rev. Thomas Hudson is an important and profound look at how human beings experience symptoms and can go behind those symptoms to find healing as whole persons. It explores the mind/body/spirit connection in new and deeper ways and offers hope to people who have unexplained medical symptoms and want to take charge of their own health. I would recommend it to professional and lay people alike."

—**James M. Long,** Minister of Pastoral Care, First Community Church, Columbus, Ohio

"This book is very easy to understand. One feels like he or she is sitting with the authors and having coffee while they explain the complex topic of hurting without an easy diagnosis and how the pace of our lives gives us many illnesses. Worth the price to hear from two very well qualified professionals."

—**Carol Langenfeld,** Dublin, Ohio

"For the reader, this book is a revelation on what physicians call *medically unexplained symptoms.* This topic is usually avoided in the typical doctor/patient relationship, so that the true impact of the problem is obscured for the general public. These authors, both highly trained professionals, have created the best written book I have read for both laymen and professionals on a little discussed but major problem of the medical profession…Not only do they reassure those suffering with pain from unexplained symptoms, they provide concrete answers and explanations of why the symptoms exist. They provide a tableau of well-considered actions that suffering patients can use to understand and relieve their pain and thereby improve their health. Highly recommended reading for both patients and doctors in providing some understanding about this often misunderstood problem."

—**Tom Krekel,** Board of Commissioners, Sanibel Public Library, Sanibel, Florida

"As healthcare becomes increasingly fragmented and user-unfriendly, quality resources for people that will help them better understand the source and significance of their symptoms so they can make appropriate decisions about which symptoms need to be pursued and by whom, are very-much needed. *Still Hurting? FIND HEALTH!* provides a comprehensive overview of the source and importance of our symptoms and provides readers with the insight and information they need to navigate the unfathomable waters of what we refer to as a healthcare system."

—**Fredric J. Pashkow, M.D., F.A.C.C., F.A.C.P.**
Co-Author of *The Women's Heart Book* and Former Editor of *Heartline* and *Cleveland Clinic Heart Advisor*

Still Hurting?
FIND HEALTH!

DISCOVER WHAT'S BEHIND YOUR
SYMPTOMS
(THAT DOCTORS CAN'T EXPLAIN)

William B. Salt II, M.D.
Thomas L. Hudson, M.Div., J.D.

Illustrations by William B. Salt II, M.D., unless otherwise credited.

Book cover and book interior layout and design by JAAD—James Arneson Art
and Design www.JaadBookDesign.com

Publisher's Cataloging-In-Publication Data
(Prepared by The Donohue Group, Inc.)

Salt, William B.

Still hurting? Find health! : discover what's behind your symptoms (that doctors
can't explain) / William B. Salt [and] Thomas L. Hudson.

   p. : ill. ; cm. -- (Still hurting? Find health! ; bk.1)

   Includes bibliographical references and index.
   ISBN: 978-0-9829612-0-9

1. Mind and body. 2. Health. 3. Stress (Physiology)--Popular works. 4. Sick--
Psychological aspects--Popular works. I. Hudson, Thomas L. II. Title. III. Title:
Discover what's behind your symptoms (that doctors can't explain)

RA776.9 .S25 2011

6132010936547

International Standard Book Number (ISBN) 978-0-9829612-0-9
Library of Congress Control Number: 2010936547

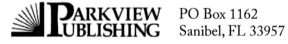

PO Box 1162
Sanibel, FL 33957

parkviewpublishing.com

For updates, more resources, and community,
visit Still Hurting? Find Health! ™ at:

stillhurtingfindhealth.com

Dedication

To everybody who hurts,
and
to our wives, Susan Salt and Cindy Hudson,
for their enduring love and support
throughout our three decades of effort
to help patients, parishioners, clients, and friends

CONTENTS

A reading guide is available on the website at:
stillhurtingfindhealth.com/Book-Club-Reading-Guide.html

Still Hurting?
FIND HEALTH!

DISCOVER WHAT'S BEHIND YOUR

SYMPTOMS

(THAT DOCTORS CAN'T EXPLAIN)

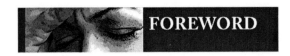

We know you're symptomatic, because everyone is. But not everyone realizes that s/he has the power to discover what's behind the symptoms to find health. Our book provides a means for this self-discovery. It contains a new model of disease and health, which is unique because it does not narrowly focus upon a single branch of knowledge to decipher why people are still hurting with symptoms that doctors can't explain. Instead, it comprehends that it is the *integration* of wisdom of ancient healing traditions, modern science, medicine, psychology, sociology, spirituality, and faith, which provides the basis for understanding why people are symptomatic and how they can find health.

In essence, we believe:

DISEASE IS DYSFUNCTION, AND SYMPTOMS ARE THE EXPRESSION.

Because

Everyone hurts. Life is hard, too fast, complicated, and very stressful; we weren't designed to live this way. The real dis-ease that results is dysfunction and the relational imbalance of our complex mind/brains, bodies, and souls, expressed as symptoms and symptom syndromes in epidemic proportion. However, by looking behind the symptoms and confronting what we find, we can regain our balance and FIND HEALTH.

The book has four parts, as shown in the illustration on the next page:

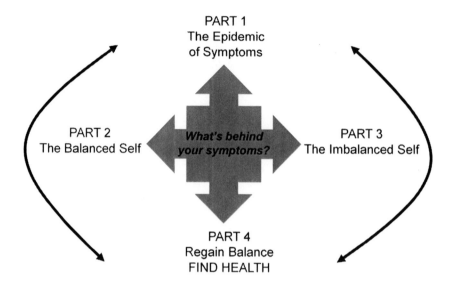

PART 1
The Epidemic
of Symptoms

PART 2
The Balanced Self

*What's behind
your symptoms?*

PART 3
The Imbalanced Self

PART 4
Regain Balance
FIND HEALTH

PART 1 describes the symptoms epidemic of which we are all a part. It then lays out the problems we face as patients and caregivers in dealing with it.

PART 2 explains how we are set up for balance and health. It describes how we are intended to function internally and in relationship to our external environment (nurture) and heredity/genetics (nature).

PART 3 describes the how and why of our becoming imbalanced, dysfunctional, and symptomatic.

PART 4 shows how we can regain our balance and function to FIND HEALTH.

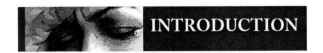
INTRODUCTION

Where do you hurt?

Which of these symptoms are yours?

What's behind them?

CHRONIC PAIN AND DISCOMFORT, SUCH AS:
Headache
Jaw pain
Facial pain
Neck pain
Back pain
Chest pain
Abdominal pain
Pelvic pain
Bladder pain
Musculoskeletal pain
Aches and pains all over

CHRONIC SYMPTOMS, SUCH AS:
Fatigue
Sleep difficulties
Bowel trouble (diarrhea, constipation, or both)
Frequent urination
Excessive weight
Enlarged waist
Lack of appetite
Weight loss
Anxiety

Depression
Obsessions
Compulsions

From these symptoms, have YOU been diagnosed by one or more specialists with any of the following symptom syndromes, also known as "functional somatic syndromes?"

GASTROENTEROLOGY: irritable bowel syndrome
(and over 30 other syndromes)

RHEUMATOLOGY: fibromyalgia syndrome

CARDIOLOGY: non-cardiac chest pain; mitral valve prolapse

PULMONOLOGY: hyperventilation; vocal cord dysfunction

GYNECOLOGY: pre-menstrual syndrome; chronic pelvic pain

INFECTIOUS DISEASE: chronic fatigue syndrome

NEUROLOGY: chronic tension headaches

OTOLARYNGOLOGY: dizziness; globus; temporomandibular joint disorder (TMJD); facial pain disorders; vocal cord dysfunction

DENTISTRY: facial pain disorders; TMJD

ALLERGY: multiple chemical sensitivity (MCS)/idiopathic environmental intolerance (IEI); multiple drug intolerance syndrome

UROLOGY: painful bladder syndrome (interstitial cystitis); painful prostate syndrome (chronic prostatitis)

SURGERY: chronic abdominal pain

ALL SPECIALTIES: multiple chemical sensitivity (MCS)/idiopathic environmental intolerance (IEI); multiple drug intolerance syndrome

There's an epidemic of pain, symptoms, and symptom syndromes!

You're not alone. Everyone hurts. Everyone needs help, at least from time to time, particularly those who feel that they have "been there, done that" but are still hurting.

Where can YOU find help?

TOO MUCH INFORMATION, NOT ENOUGH KNOWLEDGE

In a *Newsweek* article entitled, "Healthy at Any Age" (June 28 & July 5, 2010), Mary Carmichael writes,

"In the era of Google, medical advice is more confusing than ever."

You know this is true, because like most people, you seek health information from books, magazines, newspapers, and the Internet. But there is so much information available these days that it can be very difficult to know where to turn, whom to trust, and what to believe. Anyone can browse PubMed to access its over 19 million scientific papers. Yet the sheer volume of information can be overwhelming.

Furthermore, information isn't knowledge. In his play, *The Rock*, T. S. Eliot writes,

"Where is wisdom we have lost in knowledge?

Where is the knowledge we have lost in information?"

We are going to help simplify your search for knowledge.

WE CAN HELP YOU SEE CLEARLY

As a doctor and a minister, both of us have learned to ask the right questions, from which the right answers come. From familial, personal, and professional experience, we know pain and symptoms. We have spent over thirty years in caring professions in which we have assisted several hundred thousand people in their life journeys. We know that life is hard. Our patients and parishioners have testified to that. We are life-long friends and confidants who have been preparing to write this book for many years. Finally, we can offer you our integrated understanding, vision, and care-giving experience.

Firsthand, we have observed that almost everyone has either physical symptoms such as pain, discomfort, fatigue, insomnia, and/or bowel trouble, or psychological/emotional symptoms, such as anxiety, obsessions, compulsions, and depressed mood. Many have both. Some are also symptomatic in their behaviors. They don't take care of themselves. They don't eat right, and they don't exercise. Many are overweight. They smoke or drink too much. They rush through life lamenting in hindsight the *busyness* and moments lost. Some have been emotionally and physically abused.

LIFE IS HARD

In her book, *It's Always Something*, comedian Gilda Radner describes life as bittersweet. In fact, life can be downright bitter and harsh. M. Scott Peck, M.D., wrote one of the best selling self-help books of all time, *The Road Less Traveled*. The opening line reads:

"Life is difficult."

Most people would agree. What they have not recognized is the causal link between life's circumstances and their own symptoms and pain.

YOUR SYMPTOMS ARE REAL

Most symptoms that lead people to consult with doctors cannot be explained by conventional medical tests, such as blood tests, x-rays, and endoscopies. But this doesn't mean nothing's wrong. As C.S. Lewis writes:

"Pain hurts. That is what the word means."

Your symptoms are not imagined. The hurting is real.

WHAT IS BEHIND THE SYMPTOM?

Karl Menninger, the noted American psychiatrist who helped found the international psychiatric center of excellence, the Menninger Clinic, recognizes the link in his 1963 book, *The Vital Balance*. In it, he asks a profound question that we all need to ask ourselves: "What is behind the symptom?"

He asks it because he knows the importance of getting at the underlying cause of what ails us. By asking, he reiterates an age-old inquiry into the integral association of health and the relationships of body, mind, soul, and the world around us (the environment), knowing that ancient healing traditions understood that symptoms emerged when these relationships were disrupted.

Today, however, people often seek relief from symptoms without fully exploring or even ignoring the possibility that their symptoms may be indicative of disrupted body, mind, and soul relationships. They may fail to factor in the ways that they are relating to the world around them. Treatment they receive actually may aggravate the situation by also failing to explore the big relational picture regarding underlying cause. Instead, modern medicine sometimes opts for diagnostic labels and prescriptions to treat symptoms, which may or may not be medically based, without knowing what causes them.

In the healing arts, we have forgotten where we came from.

ASKING THE RIGHT QUESTIONS
TO GET THE RIGHT ANSWERS

In *The Structure of Scientific Revolutions*, his profoundly influential book on the history and philosophy of science, physicist and philosophy professor Thomas Kuhn says,

"The answers you get depend upon the questions you ask."

When it comes to getting at the truth behind your symptoms, it is critically important that you ask the right questions. Your symptoms implore you to find answers about your health, but you can't find the right answers without asking the right questions. All of us must begin by asking,

What's behind the symptoms epidemic?

The answers you get depend upon the questions you ask.

WHAT YOU CAN EXPECT BY READING OUR BOOK

After you finish this book, you will have the advantage of seeing and comprehending your health care very differently. You will understand your symptoms from a new perspective. We will help you unlearn what you have taken for granted and haven't questioned as a passive recipient of health care services. You will rediscover the power you have always had.

We will prompt you to ask the right questions about your health. We will guide and empower you so that you can find the right answers. You're going to understand what the late astronomer Carl Sagan avows:

"The absence of evidence is not evidence of absence."

You will learn to apply his words to your situation because the absence of medical evidence for the cause of your symptoms is not evidence of the absence of your very real symptoms and pain. Medical science depends upon our physical senses, mainly vision, to see. However, no one has ever seen a thought, a deeply seated emotion, or a soul. Yet, these are facets of who YOU are. There is much more to you than your mind/brain and body. The whole of you is greater than the sum of your parts. Just because all things are not evident does not mean they do not exist. You know that's true for you.

You will learn how to work with your doctors and caregivers in determining whether your symptoms can be medically explained, are medically unexplained, or both. You will know *how* your real medically unexplained symptoms happen, because they are not all in your head or imagined. You will come to understand *why* pent-up stress, emotional distress, repression, conscious and subconscious thought, doubt, and/or spiritual yearning are connected to your symptoms and consequently to your health.

You will assume responsibility for asking yourself,

What's behind my symptoms?

We will provide strategies to help you understand what you find.

HOW TO READ OUR BOOK

The book is designed for you to read through from start to finish, so resist the temptation to skip ahead. Study the format of the chapters of the first three parts:

CHAPTER TITLE lays out the essential lesson of the chapter;

QUESTIONS focus upon the content of the chapter;

QUOTES reinforce the message;

ABOUT THE QUOTES amplifies and enhances the chapter lesson;

CASE PRESENTATIONS reflect our personal, professional, and educational experience;

HEADINGS divide the chapter discussion into carefully crafted sections that build upon one another; and

LINK relates the chapter with the next chapter or part.

The format of PART 4 is a departure from the first three parts and includes HEADINGS only.

The **Bibliography** lists the sources in sequence as they are cited in each chapter.

Turn the page now to **Illustrations**, where we will introduce you to the graphics that will help you understand the lessons of our book. During your reading, we will refer you back to **Illustrations** to study them.

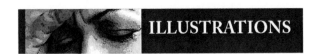

ILLUSTRATIONS

We include ten key illustrations in this section. When we discuss each graphic, we encourage you to return here for study.

FIGURE 1.1

**The Symptoms Iceberg:
An Iceberg as a Metaphor for
All of the Symptoms That People Could Experience**

Symptoms causing people to see doctors

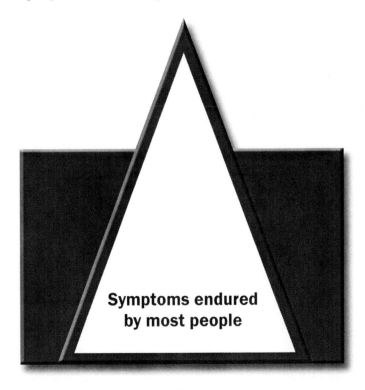

**Symptoms endured
by most people**

FIGURE 6.1

Three Potential "Causes" of the Strong Association of Symptoms with Depression and Stress

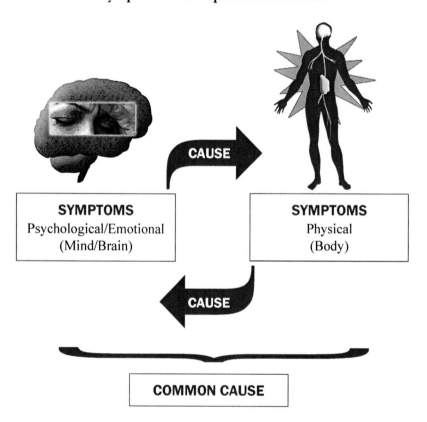

FIGURE 6.2

The Epidemic of Associated Disease, Illness, and Symptoms

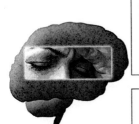

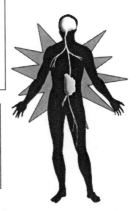

DISEASE
Depression, Anxiety
Metabolic Syndrome/Insulin Resistance, Obesity, Hypertension,
Heart, Stroke, Diabetes
Many other Diseases

ILLNESS
Depression, Anxiety
Symptom Syndromes
(e.g., IBS, Fibromyalgia)

SYMPTOMS
Psychological/Emotional
(Mind/Brain)

SYMPTOMS
Physical
(Body)

ASSOCIATION

FIGURE 10.1

The Four Major Mind/Brain Systems Involved with Feeling/Symptoms, Stress, Emotion, and Consciousness/Cognition

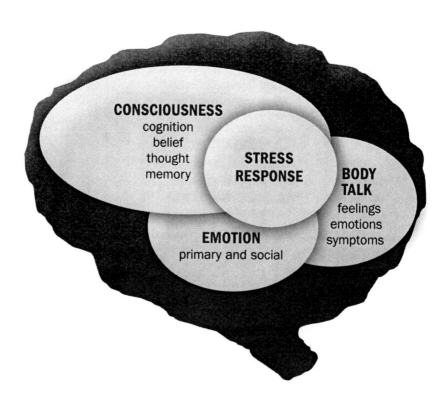

FIGURE 10.2

How YOU Emerge:

How the BODY TALK System Works

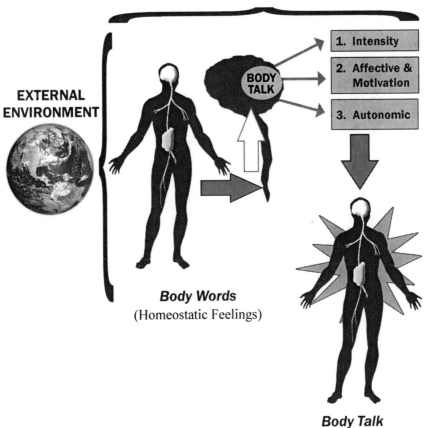

Body Words
(Homeostatic Feelings)

Body Talk
(Homeostatic Emotions)

FIGURE 13.1
Imbalance = DYSFUNCTION

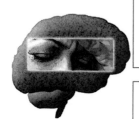

DISEASE
Depression, Anxiety
Metabolic Syndrome/Insulin Resistance, Obesity, Hypertension,
Heart, Stroke, Diabetes
Many other Diseases

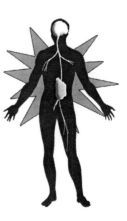

ILLNESS
Depression, Anxiety
Symptom Syndromes
(e.g., IBS, Fibromyalgia)

SYMPTOMS
Psychological/
Emotional
(Mind/Brain)

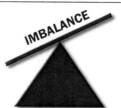

IMBALANCE

SYMPTOMS
Physical
(Body)

HOMEOSTASIS
ALLOSTASIS

DYSFUNCTION

FIGURE 13.2

A New Model of Disease:

DISEASE IS DYSFUNCTION,
AND SYMPTOMS ARE THE EXPRESSION

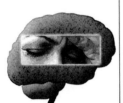

DISEASE
Depression, Anxiety
Medically Unexplained Symptoms:
Psychological/Emotional
(Mind/Brain)
Physical
(Body)
Symptom Syndromes (Medicalization)
Metabolic Syndrome/Insulin Resistance
Obesity, Hypertension, Heart, Stroke,
Diabetes, Many other Diseases

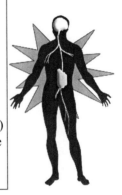

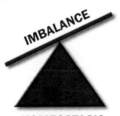

IMBALANCE

HOMEOSTASIS
ALLOSTASIS

DISEASE IS DYSFUNCTION,
AND SYMPTOMS ARE THE EXPRESSION

FIGURE 14.1

A Radio as a Metaphor for
DYSFUNCTION of the BODY TALK System:

How YOU Are Symptomatic with SYMPTOMS
(Medically Unexplained Symptoms)

and SYMPTOM SYNDROMES
(Central Sensitivity Syndromes/Functional Somatic Syndromes)

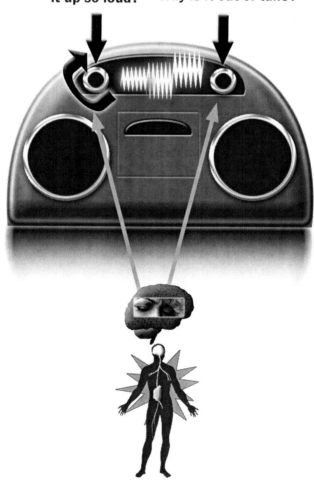

FIGURE 14.2

Complexity Interrelationships

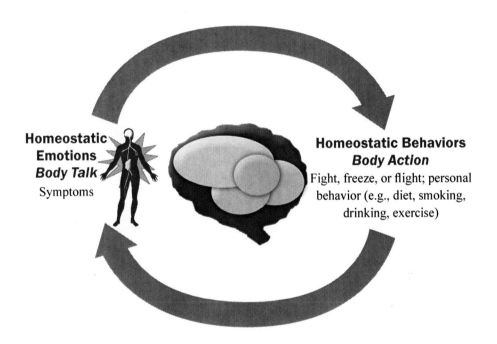

Homeostatic Emotions
Body Talk
Symptoms

Homeostatic Behaviors
Body Action
Fight, freeze, or flight; personal behavior (e.g., diet, smoking, drinking, exercise)

FIGURE YOU.1

See Differently:
DYSFUNCTION (Imbalance) and
STRESS, EMOTION, CONSCIOUSNESS, SOUL, & BEHAVIOR

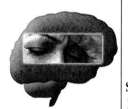

DISEASE
Depression, Anxiety
Medically Unexplained Symptoms:
Psychological/Emotional
(Mind/Brain)
Physical
(Body)
Symptom Syndromes (Medicalization)
Metabolic Syndrome/Insulin Resistance
Obesity, Hypertension, Heart, Stroke,
Diabetes, Many other Diseases

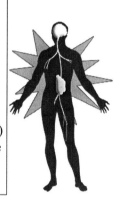

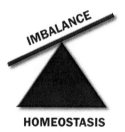

IMBALANCE

HOMEOSTASIS
ALLOSTASIS

STRESS, EMOTION, CONSCIOUSNESS, SOUL & BEHAVIOR

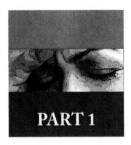

PART 1

The Epidemic of Symptoms

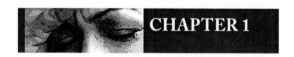

CHAPTER 1

YOU Are Symptomatic

QUESTIONS

Am I the only one who's hurting?

What's causing my symptoms?

QUOTE

"What is behind the symptom?"

The Vital Balance (1963)
KARL MENNINGER, M.D. (Psychiatrist, Founder Menninger Clinic)

ABOUT THE QUOTE

You're looking for answers. Often you don't realize how important it is to ask the right questions to find the right answers. This is especially true when you hurt. Questions you don't ask can influence your health outcomes. By the way, did you notice that the title of the book begins with a question?

CASE PRESENTATION

It's three A.M.

The rain has stopped, but your mind hasn't. From family matters to finances, from job to health, it keeps replaying topics better left for the clarity of sunlight. For the moment, the neighbor's pocket-sized dog has ceased its yipping. Something, though, keeps yipping and nipping at you. Restless legs—you fidget, no matter how many pillows you put under your knees. The knots in your neck and shoulders really hurt.

Tossing side to side, you hear and feel the thumping of your heart against the therapeutic pillow. The thump is coming from near your ear! That's scary, so you have to shift positions to make it go away. Getting up, you stretch, tighten, and loosen your legs to try to get them to relax. Off balance, you trip going to the bathroom. You drink a glass of water, lie back down, and close your eyes. They pop back open as you start wondering why you've felt so crummy lately.

Is something wrong?

Alarm set for six, it is now four A.M., but you are not asleep; you're sweating and asking questions. You promise yourself to call and make an appointment for a check-up.

Several weeks later, you finally have the opportunity to consult with your doctor. You're anxious for many reasons, not the least of which is your silent observation that,

The waiting room is filled with patients!

Taking a seat, you wonder how long it's going to be before it's your turn. You're impatient and restless as you ponder how your symptoms will be diagnosed and treated. You know how off-kilter you are and quietly ask yourself,

When did life get so hard? When did I begin to feel this lousy?

Like that silly nursery rhyme that no one ever bothered to explain, you're beginning to feel like a shell of your old self. Like Humpty Dumpty, you're on edge and fragile. Sometimes it's the headaches. Occasionally (but by your count more frequently), you have palpitations, rapid heartbeat, and quick shooting pains in your shoulder. You have experienced tingling and numbness in your hands and feet. Your back and neck muscles are knotted up. Low back pain puts you on the floor. As one of those people whose tension turns inward to the gut, you get stomach cramps, heartburn, or acid reflux no over-the-counter drug can touch, no matter what the ads claim. One recent reflux episode felt like a heart attack. You're more tired than usual. Poor sleep is certainly a culprit, but something else is going on. You used to have more energy and pep. Now, you're fatigued and feel a vague *dis-ease* that you can't quite put your finger on, let alone name. It adds to the constant stress and weighs you down. Flipping through old copies of *Good Housekeeping or Golf Digest*, still waiting for the nurse to call your name, your mind again rewinds to other pressing matters. Family life or work has been difficult. Perhaps more aggressive and energetic types are taking bites out of your memos, ideas, and paycheck. Maybe you find yourself beginning to parent your parents and you keep rehearsing what you need to say to them. While rehearsing, you remember times, moments, memories you'd rather bury or forget. You remember and get upset because you feel the need to accommodate, please, and be accepted by them. But you keep that to yourself. Funny, on that score, how you've been accommodating and trying to please others since you were a kid. As old tapes replay in your head, the door opens, and the nurse glances your way.

"The doctor will see you now."

You run a checklist on aches and pains as you head down the corridor to exam room #6. As you follow the nurse, you think,

I hope I can remember what I want to tell the doctor.

That's why you're here. You are here to describe those symptoms. Though they sorely stress you, the problems in the rest of your life will have to wait. Even if you are inclined to discuss them, you won't have the time. You may not even get through your symptoms list before the doctor sizes up what you say and walks out the door with your chart. Those other patients— with multiple symptoms—wait. The doctor knows a long workday awaits and scurries from one patient to the next.

Your health care is time-managed, and your doctor is on the clock.

Between the two of you, much will remain unspoken.

It gets worse.

PROBLEMS THE CASE PRESENTATION RAISES

The symptoms you can't put into words will go begging for evaluation. Those you do describe may get a name or label that may not be indicative of the real problem. You might not want or be able to discuss major stress issues in your life. Regardless, your doctor lacks the time and perhaps the inclination to listen. You may leave the office with a diagnosis and prescription, yet be no wiser or nearer to symptom/cause interconnection than you were before.

This time-constrained interaction between you and your doctor is frustrating, unsatisfactory, and bad for your health. The reasons for it are overtly and subtly multi-faceted. At root is a fragmented and inadequate understanding of personal health care.

A SUMMARY OF WHAT'S GOING ON IN THE WORLD OF MODERN HEALTH CARE

→ Everyone hurts.
→ Time with doctors is increasingly limited.
→ Medical science is imperfect.
→ Medicine is both art and science.
→ Few understand that the whole is greater than the sum of its parts.
→ Care of the person is increasingly fragmented from within (with multiple symptoms that are seemingly unrelated) and without (multiple doctors and caregivers seemingly not relating with one another).
→ *Medicalization* ("the invocation of a medical diagnosis explaining symptoms without evidence of disease and the application of medical intervention to treat them") is widespread.
→ The patient/doctor relationship is threatened by multiple influences.
→ Many people do not trust doctors.
→ The individual must be responsible for his/her health.

Life is perplexing, arduous, and very stressful. You weren't biologically designed to live it this way, so you're symptomatic. Even if it isn't apparent to you, this is the way it is for everybody. You are not alone.

YOU ARE PART OF A WORLDWIDE EPIDEMIC

This epidemic involves everyone with interrelated, uncomfortable, distressing, and commonly painful bodily and psychological symptoms that interfere with life, relationships, and work. When these symptoms are recurrent and ongoing, people consult with doctors, but when medical tests fail to explain them, they are called *medically unexplained symptoms (MUS)*. Furthermore, doctors describe and diagnose collections of symptoms as *symptom syndromes*. They call them *functional somatic syndromes*, which include irritable bowel syndrome, fibromyalgia syndrome, and psychiatric syndromes (depression and anxiety). Many patients have seen several doctors and received more than one diagnosis. While most of these symptoms and syndromes are not life threatening, two syndromes are potential killers: depression and the metabolic syndrome (also known as metabolic syndrome X and insulin resistance syndrome). While the symptoms of metabolic syndrome are often explainable by tests and, therefore, not always classified as MUS, we include the syndrome because of its strong association and overlap with MUS syndromes. Note as well that doctors often associate and diagnose depression and/or stress as the cause of physical symptoms that cannot be explained.

SICK OF SYMPTOMS

A National Institute of Mental Health-funded study published in the *Archives of General Psychiatry* finds that:

"More than half of U.S. adults have a physical or mental condition that prevents them from working or conducting their usual duties for several days each year."

Among those adults, each experienced an average of over a month of disability per year. Nationwide, this adds up to 3.7 billion disability days per year! Musculoskeletal disorders, especially back and neck pain, were responsible for the greatest number of disability days (1.2 billion), while major depression caused the second greatest number of disability days (387 million). Dr. Kathleen Merikangas, the lead author of the study says, "These figures suggest an enormous burden on the people who have one or more of these conditions, their families and their employers."

THE SYMPTOMS ICEBERG

In an important medical study published in 1987, "Exploring the Iceberg—Common Symptoms and How People Care for Them," Doctors Verbrugge and Ascione explain that most people endure their symptoms and don't consult with doctors. In the **Illustrations** section, Figure 1.1 shows an iceberg as a metaphor for all of the symptoms that people could experience. Everyone has symptoms at one time or another and many people are chronically symptomatic, yet the bulk of the Symptoms Iceberg is submerged, indicating that most people endure their symptoms without seeking medical care. These symptoms are considered mild and harmless. Some people do decide to consult with doctors about their symptoms, as depicted by the smaller portion of the Symptoms Iceberg visible above the water line. These symptoms are considered distressing and/or potentially serious.

The most common symptom occasioning consultation is pain. While there is nothing imaginary about the symptoms, most have little or no physical explanation for them.

This you will fully come to appreciate as we refer to the Symptoms Iceberg again in Chapter 4.

THE DOCTOR PATIENT RELATIONSHIP

The mass of the Symptoms Iceberg is an immense navigational problem in health care. Compounding the difficulty is the tension inherent in the doctor-patient relationship. Given the fragmentary nature of the diagnostic process, patients, doctors, and other care-giving professionals can become disconnected, confused, and frustrated. Many people consult with multiple doctors and caregivers in seeking diagnosis and relief from symptoms.

Research confirms that doctors experience one in every six primary care visits as difficult.

Dr. Kurt Kroenke comments in a February 23, 2009 editorial in the *Archives of General Internal Medicine* that "studies in this area had a somewhat pejorative perspective on the 'difficult patient' and included labels such as 'black holes' or 'heartsink' in the United Kingdom and 'difficult,' 'problem,' 'disliked,' 'frustrating,' 'troublesome,' or even 'hateful' in the United States." The difficulty is more recently attributed to patient and doctor interrelation factors. The mutual distress in these difficult encounters is real. Doctors' mindsets contribute to the difficulty, especially when patients present psychological symptoms or disorders (e.g., depression, anxiety, and substance abuse) and/or multiple medically unexplained symptoms.

Frankly, most doctors don't particularly like to see patients with medically unexplained symptoms, because they are unable or unwilling to provide them with answers and explanations.

You're symptomatic with these medically unexplained symptoms. Everyone is.

ASKING THE RIGHT QUESTIONS TO GET THE RIGHT ANSWERS

Your symptoms urge you to find answers about your health, but you can't find the right answers without asking the right questions. Unfortunately, you are at the great disadvantage of not knowing the right questions to ask because of major shortcomings and one huge change in the health care system. Some of the shortcomings have been briefly described before and will be detailed throughout the book. The huge change in health care deserves some explanation now.

THE DISADVANTAGE OF *MEDICALIZATION*

During the past several decades, caregivers and care recipients have been both the beneficiaries and unwitting victims of a significant transformation in the interplay between daily life problems and health care management. The term used for this change is *medicalization*, which is the process by which problems that may not be medically based become defined and treated as medical problems, usually in terms of symptom illnesses, syndromes, and disorders.

Particularly nebulous in the *medicalization* transformation are the roles of physician and patient.

In the delivery of health care, doctors continue to be pivotal in diagnosing symptoms and recommending treatment. They order tests, make referrals to their professional peer group's specialists, and write prescriptions for their patients. Yet their position as the preeminent authorities on prescriptive treatment is now being challenged and often compromised by advertising campaigns aimed directly at the health care consumer. Pharmaceutical ads saturate print media and the airwaves. The ads advise readers and viewers about the benefits of using certain products to alleviate what they once thought of as daily life problems and realities, but are now to consider as medical conditions. Sadness, social anxiety, menopause, insomnia, and low libido are a few examples advertisers use to tie the consumer's particular "medical condition" to their named product, the point of which is to teach the reader/viewer to ask for the product by name. Armed with this knowledge, the patient now has the prescriptive remedy to give the doctor.

Lost in all of this is that nowhere is anyone asking, "What's behind the symptom?"

Instead, the ad emphasis is on the drug, remedy, and quick fix. In the appeal to the consumer patient, *right answers* abound. What is missing is the need to ask the right questions, especially Dr. Menninger's question.

MEDICALIZATION INCREASES DEMAND FOR HEALTH CARE

In his book, *The Medicalization of Society: On the Transformation of Human Conditions into Treatable Disorders*, medical sociologist Peter Conrad addresses the multiple illnesses, syndromes, psychological states, and behaviors that now receive medical diagnosis and medical treatment. He asks,

"Does it mean that a whole range of life's problems have now received medical diagnoses and are subject to medical treatment, despite dubious evidence of their medical nature?"

Medicalization increases the demand for medical service by increasing the number of symptoms that are evaluated medically, and by increasing patients' expectations of medical help and hopefully, cure. This enlarges the

Symptoms Iceberg and its exposed tip and puts you and your doctor at a great disadvantage. Now you both must discern between physical and/or psychological/emotional symptoms that are part of the human condition and those that reflect true medical disorders. Having to discern the difference makes finding what's behind the symptoms that much more difficult. Meanwhile, you are still asking,

Why am I still hurting and symptomatic?

While you see that you are not alone and that you are not imagining your symptoms, you wonder what's wrong.

LINK

To empower you with the ability to answer this question, we will begin on a personal note in the next chapter by presenting you with our own case studies.

CHAPTER 2

We (the Authors) Are Symptomatic, Too

QUESTION

You're a doctor and you're a minister; are you saying that you both suffer with distressing symptoms, just as I do?

QUOTES

"I have a bad back."

DR. BILL SALT (Before the "Big Aha!")

"I'm going to see a doctor about my neck.
I hope I don't need another operation.
I better bring up the heart symptoms, too."

REV. TOM HUDSON (Before the "Big Aha!")

ABOUT THE QUOTES

Both of us have learned hard lessons about the relationship between stressful work and personal health. We believe that medical schools and seminaries, on behalf of their students, should consider including in their orientation guides the following quotation from Thomas Jefferson in a letter written to Thomas Mann Randolph, Jr., July 6, 1787:

With your talents and industry, with science, and that steadfast honesty which eternally pursues right, regardless of consequences, you may promise yourself everything but health, without which there is no happiness. An attention to health then should take the place of every other object. The time necessary to secure this by active exercises, should be devoted to it in preference to every other pursuit.

CASE PRESENTATION: THE DOCTOR

I am Bill Salt, a sixty-three-year-old M.D. (gastroenterologist), and one of the subjects of this chapter. I present you with my own case because I can't think of a better way to help you see that we are all involved in this epidemic together, whether we are conscious of it or not.

I began having back pain while I was in medical school. First, I experienced intermittent episodes of acute low back pain that were often associated with sports activities such as basketball and touch football. They didn't last very long, and I wasn't particularly upset by them. Athletes are used to having a variety of aches, pains, and injuries. But the attacks started to come more frequently with less strenuous activity and began to last longer, often for several weeks or more. My back was stiff and inflexible between attacks, but I was still sort of okay with it.

Then, around age forty, I ruptured a disc in my low back—a diagnosis confirmed by magnetic resonance imaging (MRI). It required I miss work (a first) and involved a prolonged convalescence. The pain became chronic, and I became convinced that I had a bad back and would never really get over the problem. I feared that any unpredictable movement would cause an attack and set me back for weeks. I now realize that I was depressed at times. I felt sorry for myself because it just didn't seem right that I had to work so hard being a doctor totally devoted to patients while having painful and distressing symptoms. I resigned myself to chronic pain and having to set limits on my activities. I didn't miss any more work, but I often missed other activities so I could lie down and rest my bad back. I *backed out* of social obligations at the last minute, leaving my wife to cover for me. I couldn't throw the ball or play sports with my children. I quit playing basketball, my favorite sport, as well as golf. All this put a strain on my family.

Eventually, I consulted with a good friend and colleague, Dr. Ed Season, a specialist in musculoskeletal medicine and surgery, who convinced me that I could recover and heal. He taught me that back pain is complex and involves much more than structural problems, such as a disc herniation or rupture. Most of the time, back pain cannot be explained by medical tests. Later, ironically, Ed himself hurt with a herniated disc in his back, from which he completely recovered without surgery. He knew he would eventually, but he suffered for months. I came to understand that my back problem was related to a combination of factors:

→ I had gradually become overweight since medical school. I graduated from high school at around 160 pounds and eventually weighed around 200 pounds. Incidentally, I'm a little over 6 feet, 3 inches tall.
→ I was not in good physical condition.
→ My back pain was associated with stress, emotional distress, and negative beliefs and thoughts, even though I was not consciously aware of it.
→ The illness adversely affected my entire well-being: physical, psychological, emotional, and spiritual.
→ I didn't really get better until I realized how unconscious about all of this I had been and developed a self-care plan, which included better health-related beliefs and behaviors.

I felt pretty good about my back until I developed a new symptom. Around the age of fifty, I began to notice widespread discomfort and pain associated with fatigue and poor sleep, which were often the consequences of work stress. This occurred when I was on call in the hospital for a week at a time. During these difficult weeks, I worked anywhere from seventy-five to ninety-five hours. Many nights, sleep was disrupted by phone calls that necessitated my going back to the hospital to take care of people with digestive emergencies, such as internal bleeding. It felt like having a hangover. The symptoms got worse as the week progressed and did not improve or resolve until I had recovered over the following weekend.

During my professional career, I became increasingly conscious of how irritable, withdrawn, and cranky I could be when work stress accumulated. Of course, my wife of forty years knows about what I am sharing, and I am grateful for her love, support, and acceptance throughout my career. Later in the book, I'll tell you about changes I've made in my life, and especially about what happened after I developed a new symptom.

TRANSITION

In ministry, as in medicine, professional caregivers have to be willing to give themselves away. They are on call twenty-four hours a day. They are approached in grocery aisles, drug stores, and restaurants by people with problems and symptoms who want help and diagnosis. Their homes are extensions of their offices. They know they can't meet everybody's needs and expectations, yet it nags at them when they don't or can't. The burdens they carry and the knowledge they have of others' personal lives weigh heavily upon them.

The stress builds up. They don't vent very well.

They become symptomatic.

CASE PRESENTATION: THE MINISTER/ATTORNEY

I am Tom Hudson, a sixty-two-year-old who has served for over thirty years as a minister and legal counselor and teacher. As the second case presenter, I agree with my friend, Bill Salt, that a good way to link our symptomatic tales is to tell you mine.

During the latter stages of serving as senior minister of a large metropolitan church, I began having a variety of physical symptoms that for several months I kept to myself:

→ My heart began pounding sporadically, like a fist jabbing me from the inside out.

→ My neck and shoulders hurt and became increasingly stiff.

→ My left hand and foot tingled; the foot itself was often numb.

I hoped over time and a week's vacation that the symptoms would go away. They didn't. After a few weeks back at work, they grew worse. The neck pain, tingling, and numbness became constant. I had low back surgery a few years before and knew first-hand the nerve-related symptoms. Whether the tingling and numbness were phantom remnants of previous damage or symptoms of a new problem, I didn't know. What I did know was that I did not want to undergo another operation. My neck really hurt.

The heart thump was another matter. The punch became harder and more constant. It scared me. My fear triggered more jabs. I had to deal with what was happening. I made an appointment with our family internist. He and his staff listened attentively as I described my symptoms. I will never forget the keen listening and observation skills of the nurse practitioner Jennifer O'Brien. (Thank you, Jennifer, wherever you are.) The heart issues led to a stress test, ECG, MRI, and my wearing for six weeks a recording device that monitored the thump. It had four electrodes that I hooked up daily to my skin and a recorder I attached to my belt. At work, I passed it off as a pager. When the contractions came, I recorded them and sent them by phone for evaluation. After weeks of monitoring, doctors confirmed the MRI results. The punches and jabs were PACs (premature atrial contractions). My heart was misfiring. To regulate the spark, I went on a beta-blocker.

The neck pain continued. I was referred back to Dr. William Miely, the orthopedic surgeon who had previously operated on me. His office performed extensive nerve tests on my arms and legs and eventually ordered an MRI. Two MRIs in two months on two different sets of symptoms—I thought I was falling apart! I was worried when I returned to Dr. Miely's office for the MRI results. To his credit, he sat with me and discussed them. Six upper spinal and neck discs were disintegrating and arthritic, but he wasn't going to cut. I was stunned and relieved. Instead, he discussed how much he and his peers were learning about the impact of life and work stressors upon the spine, muscles, and nerves. From previous conversations around my surgery, he knew what I did for a living and the size of the church I served. From what he had heard from his own minister friends, he suggested that basic changes were in order. They had to do with setting boundaries, honoring self-care, and lowering stress.

I faced a dilemma. I didn't know how to work at any other pace. What drove me to serve well also made me vulnerable. What a paradox! My strengths were my weaknesses. If I kept going the way I had been, I was going to be in deep trouble. Given the issues with my health, I decided to retire from parish ministry and concentrate on writing and teaching part-time.

Several months after retiring from the church I served, my neck pain lessened. While the tingling and numbness in my left leg and foot is an occasional reminder of past nerve damage, my heart has returned to a regular beat. I do occasional teaching now and enjoy friends, family, and two grandsons. I've developed better boundaries, and I am not as stressed as I was before. In my life, symptoms were warning signs. Fortunately, I received the kind of care that medicine, at its best, has to offer. I am also more aware of taking responsibility for my own health.

OUR BIG AHA!

These case presentations describe our "Big Aha!" experiences. Each of us learned hard lessons about the causes and meaning of our symptoms. Continuing to learn from experience, we want to share our discoveries with you.

LEARNING THE HARD WAY

Symptoms have meaning. The meaning is not what you may think it is. Most people believe there must be a direct medical cause of their symptoms that can be identified through tests. You will soon learn that this is not the case. It is true that some symptoms signal the presence of a potentially serious and/or medically treatable problem, and we will address two very important symptom complexes in this book: depression and metabolic syndrome.

However, the amazing fact is that most symptoms remain medically unexplained!

By the time that you have finished this book, you will discover what's behind them. You will see how symptoms are generated, why they happen, and how you can help yourself when you are symptomatic.

LINK

The next chapter discusses the pain and symptom epidemic and defines the medical language and terminology that doctors use in their description of symptoms.

CHAPTER 3

There's a Symptom Epidemic, and We're All in It

QUESTION

Does everybody have symptoms and decide to see a doctor about them?

QUOTE

"Symptoms are a regular part of the human experience."

"Symptoms: In the Head or in the Brain?"

Annals of Internal Medicine, 2001
ANTHONY L. KOMAROFF, M.D.

ABOUT THE QUOTE

In May 2001, Dr. Anthony Komaroff, Harvard Medical School professor of medicine and editor-in-chief of Harvard Health Publications, wrote an article in supplement to the prestigious medical journal, *Annals of Internal Medicine,* devoted entirely to the medical investigation of symptoms. The title of his article, "Symptoms: In the Head or in the Brain?" implicates the mind/brain's involvement with symptoms that are manifestations of the life experience.

CASE PRESENTATION

I am sixty-three years of age and at least sixty pounds heavier than I was when I graduated in 1965 from Bexley High School in Columbus, Ohio, where Dr. Salt and I were classmates and friends. Still good friends, he has asked me to describe any symptoms I have.

I have intermittent headaches, which I either ignore and endure or self-treat with acetaminophen or ibuprofen that I buy at the drug store without prescription. I also have low back pain now and then, but it doesn't interfere with my work or my life. Sometimes it gets kind of bad, but I get by. Now that I think about it, I probably feel more tired than I should and good sleep seems harder to get. I have always been a little constipated, but about once or twice a month, I have attacks of cramping abdominal pain associated with diarrhea. I don't think I have any serious medical problems, so I haven't consulted a doctor about any of these things. I have been meaning to lose weight and get into shape without much success.

SYMPTOMS ARE PART OF EVERYBODY'S LIFE

John Sarno, M.D., is professor of rehabilitative medicine at New York University Hospital and the author of *The Mind/Body Prescription: Healing the Body, Healing the Pain,* and *The Divided Mind: The Epidemic of Mind-Body Disorders.* He says,

"There is an epidemic of pain and symptoms."

He's right. It's a huge epidemic. And it's complicated.

A classic medical study of over one million men and women conducted in the 1960s by Dr. E.C. Hammond showed that at any moment, at least half of everyone in the study admitted to headaches and more than one-third admitted to fatigue. From current medical data, one-third of healthy people will have aches and pains in their muscles at any given time, and one-fifth will report significant fatigue. Nearly ninety percent of the population report at least one bodily symptom, such as headache, joint ache, muscle stiffness, or diarrhea in any two-to-four week period. A typical adult has one such symptom every four to six days.

A medical study published in 2000 by Dr. Robert Sandler and colleagues from the University of North Carolina confirms that forty percent of the people in the study have at least one digestive symptom, such as abdominal pain, diarrhea, or constipation every month. Most people rated their symptoms as moderate to severe in intensity and reported that they caused some limitations in their daily activities.

CHILDREN AND ADOLESCENTS ARE NOT IMMUNE

According to Joshua Lipsitz, Ph.D., assistant clinical professor of psychology at Columbia University College of Physicians and Surgeons, approximately one in twenty child and adolescent visits to pediatricians and family physicians are for physical symptoms that have no medical explanation.

The most common symptoms of children and adolescents are recurrent abdominal pain and headaches.

A 2009 study in the *Journal of Child Neurology* finds that over a twelve month period, 17.1% of children reported frequent or severe headaches. Based upon a community-based survey reported in *Clinical Gastroenterology and Hepatology*, German researchers show that over a three month period, more than one-third of the children ages three to ten years and more than one-fourth of adolescents between the ages of eleven to seventeen suffer recurrent abdominal pain. Many of these young people consult with doctors, and the authors of the study conclude that abdominal pain is "an important public health problem in children and adolescents." Dr. Lipsitz also finds that recurrent chest pain accounts for more than 600,000 office visits annually in the United States by individuals ages ten to twenty-one. Researchers from Denmark, reporting in July 2009 in the *European Journal of Epidemiology*, have also found that medically unexplained symptoms are common health complaints in five to seven-year-old children. The most common symptoms are limb pain, headache, and abdominal pain.

SYMPTOMS ARE WORLD WIDE

Having symptoms is not unique to Americans. While cultural differences influence what symptoms are expressed, everybody is symptomatic throughout the world. For example, Norwegian researchers led by C. Ihlebaek, writing in the *Scandinavian Journal of Public Health*, report that "subjective health complaints are very common in the normal population."

The language, "subjective health complaints," is equivalent to *medically unexplained symptoms (MUS)*.

In European and North American studies, chronic pain affects between twelve percent and thirty-five percent of the population at any time and between forty-nine percent and eighty percent across the life span. Turkish physician, Dr. K. Sayar, writes about medically unexplained symptoms in the medical journal *Turk Psikiyatri Derg* and describes the bodily symptoms associated with depression, which is a very important observation that we will discuss throughout this book. Furthermore, a recent study in the *International Journal of Behavioral Medicine* confirms that musculoskeletal complaints, fatigue, mood changes, and gastrointestinal complaints are not limited to industrialized societies.

SYMPTOMS ENDURED

As discussed in Chapter 1, even though everybody is symptomatic at one time or another, most people tolerate their symptoms without seeking medical consultation.

Studies show that only about one in four people with symptoms decides to consult health care professionals, but symptoms are what prompt people to see the doctor.

Why people seek diagnosis and relief and what happens when they do is the subject of **PART 1** of this book.

HOW DOCTORS EVALUATE SYMPTOMS

Initially, we are going to introduce to you the medical language and terminology that doctors use to describe, classify, and diagnose symptoms. This will help you understand how doctors approach patients symptomatic with disease and illness. You also need to understand the questions doctors ask patients and themselves. What they ask and why will help you comprehend physician/patient interaction and enable you to better formulate your own questions and concerns.

Symptoms and/or Signs?

Patients tell doctors about their symptoms and signs. Doctors cannot see the symptoms. They hear them described as pain or fatigue. In contrast, signs are visible and evident. Examples of signs include fever, rapid pulse, or a lump the physician can feel. Suffice it to say, doctors have a greater comfort level evaluating signs than listening to descriptions of symptoms. What doctors can see is evident to them and therefore trustworthy, but what a patient perceives and tries to describe is nebulous, at best, to the doctor.

Disease and/or Illness?

In 1977, in the *Medical Clinics of North America*, Dr. A. Reading clarifies the definitions of and distinctions between **disease** and **illness**. The difference is a key component in understanding how doctors evaluate your symptoms.

Disease is the manifestation of a pathological state that is externally verifiable. This means the condition can be detected by medical tests. For example, duodenal ulcer—a disease—is confirmed by an endoscopic examination.

On the other hand, doctors view *illness* as a patient's perception of poor health, pain, and impaired ability to function. Illness is evident to doctors by the patient's:

→ Symptom reports: "Doctor, I'm in pain."
→ Illness beliefs: "I'm sick and there's something wrong with my stomach!"
→ Illness behavior: "I can't even go to the store, let alone work."

It's easy to understand *disease with illness*. An example of disease with illness is an individual with a duodenal ulcer causing abdominal pain.

It's not so easy to understand *disease without illness*. A person can have a duodenal ulcer without any pain at all. WBS has seen this hundreds of times when called in to help a patient who suddenly vomits blood, the cause of which is a bleeding duodenal ulcer.

But the hardest case scenario remains. It's the mystery of *illness without disease*. Here we have symptoms and illness without disease, because medical tests fail to show a cause. This causes the greatest misunderstanding between doctor and patient—the mystery of illness without disease, of symptoms without cause (medically unexplained symptoms)—and is the main subject of this book.

Serious or Self-Limited?

The first diagnostic consideration is whether the symptom or symptoms could indicate the presence of disease that may be serious and potentially life threatening, such as chest pain, indicating a heart attack, or abdominal pain signaling an inflamed gall bladder. The alternative consideration is whether the symptom or symptoms reflect the presence of a non-serious condition—what doctors call *self-limited*. This term means that symptoms are harmless, expected to resolve on their own, and either require no treatment or only treatment to facilitate recovery or relieve them. An example of self-limited symptoms would be a viral upper respiratory tract infection, known as the common cold.

Acute or Chronic?

Next, doctors consider whether the symptoms are acute or chronic, either of which may be serious. Acute symptoms have a sudden onset that can occur immediately or over several hours. Chronic symptoms are persistent and last for weeks, months, or years. Chronic and recurring symptoms are known as *relapsing* when they occur repeatedly.

Medically Explained or Medically Unexplained?

Along with considering the seriousness of symptoms, their acuity, and potential resolution, doctors also assess whether the cause of the symptom or symptoms can be confirmed with medical studies. Study examples include blood tests, X-rays, imaging scans, and endoscopic examinations (e.g. colonoscopy). When medical tests confirm the cause, physicians consider symptoms to be medically explained symptoms, which are examples of disease with illness. The medical term for cause is *etiology*. For example, pneumonia might be the etiology or cause of a patient's shortness of breath, chest pain, and fever.

If the cause for symptoms is not found after careful evaluation, doctors will often simply take note of and describe the patient's symptom or symptoms. For example, the symptom of muscle pain without a clear cause would be labeled as *myalgia* (muscle pain) or *myalgia NOS* (not otherwise specified). Even when a doctor uses this label, it is still possible that a serious disease or disorder will occasionally declare itself and be diagnosed in time. Typically, however, the doctor's indication implies that the symptom or symptoms are either self-limited or, if they become persistent and/or recurrent, are not life threatening.

On charts and patient records, doctors may use the term *idiopathic* to describe symptoms that are not attributable to a specific medical cause. They use the term when there is no explanation for the symptoms. Doctors often place this diagnostic term before the symptom, description, or syndrome. Muscle pain of unknown etiology would be labeled as *idiopathic myalgia* or as *myalgia of unknown etiology*.

Most symptoms are not accounted for by medical testing.

In a 2007 medical article entitled "Classification and Diagnosis of Patients with Medically Unexplained Symptoms" in the *Journal of General Internal Medicine*, Michigan State University doctors reinforce the point that:

Symptoms prompting the sufferer to seek health care, but which lack causal confirmation even after medical evaluation, are called *medically unexplained symptoms*, or *MUS*.

Most medically unexplained symptoms are manifestations of **illness without disease**.

Functional?

Among themselves, doctors also use the term *functional* to describe medically unexplained symptoms not considered manifestations of a potentially serious disease. The term is often used by doctors when tests fail to show a specific medical cause.

Functional means that the symptom is related to a problem with the way the body works and functions.

For example, when medical tests used to evaluate abdominal pain associated with altered bowel function (diarrhea, constipation, or both) are normal, a doctor may diagnose a functional gastrointestinal disorder, such as irritable bowel syndrome. When a person has generalized body pain associated with fatigue and insomnia, a doctor may diagnose a functional rheumatologic disorder, such as fibromyalgia syndrome. While you may run across the term functional in the health care reading that you do, you won't often hear your doctor use it. Why is this?

Functional is a code word used by the medical community.

Since there's no time to explain the meaning of the word, it's included in the chart but usually not in the discussion with the patient. As will be discussed in Chapter 5, the term *functional* is often tied to the usage of another code word—*syndrome*. Used together, these code terms usually mean that doctors stop looking for any alternative explanation or cause. They stop looking behind the symptoms.

Psychosomatic?

Another term applied to functional medically unexplained symptoms is *psychosomatic*. Broken down into its two parts, it includes *psyche*, meaning mind or soul, and *soma*, meaning body. Doctors usually avoid the psychosomatic label because it has developed a negative connotation, being erroneously associated with mental illness or delusion, which adds further injury to the sufferer.

We emphasize three facts about medically unexplained symptoms:

→ Most chronic ongoing or recurrent symptoms are medically unexplained.

→ Most medically unexplained physical symptoms are considered functional.

→ Medically unexplained symptoms are *real* and not *"all in the head,"* as you know from your experience.

Moreover, as explained below, medically unexplained symptoms are classified as either physical (somatic) or psychological (emotional).

Physical (Somatic) Medically Unexplained Symptoms?

These are bodily symptoms of distress that are uncomfortable or worrisome. They are usually called physical by doctors who mainly care for patients with medical disorders and *somatic* by mental health specialists. These two terms are similar, and they will be used interchangeably in this book.

Physical symptoms and physical disorders (i.e. medical disorders where the etiology [cause] is established) are not equivalent. Many patients with physical symptoms, such as back pain, do not have a medical disorder, such as osteoarthritis, which would account for the presence and/or severity of the symptom. Many patients with medical disorders have no symptoms; for example, the patient with osteoarthritis seen on x-ray may have no back pain at all.

Listing all the symptoms that people can experience would be overwhelming here, but looking at how doctors commonly place symptoms into two groups will be helpful.

Constitutional/Vital Symptoms

These symptoms reflect disturbances of an overall sense of well-being, good health, and function. Examples include lack of energy and fatigue, change in appetite (the term *anorexia* refers to loss of appetite), change in weight, nausea (this symptom does not always mean a problem in the digestive system), sleep disturbance, and sexual dysfunction (most commonly, low sexual interest or low libido).

Have you ever noticed that your energy and appetite can be affected by stress and emotional distress and that your weight can fluctuate?

System Symptoms

The typical way to classify symptoms is to attribute them to the main body organ system that seems to be involved. The most common systems are gastrointestinal, musculoskeletal (rheumatologic), urogenital (urologic and gynecologic), and autonomic (nervous).

Gastrointestinal System

The digestive tract or gut is approximately thirty feet in length. Many different symptoms can occur from the top (throat) to the bottom (rectum and anus). Some of the most common symptoms include throat discomfort, chest pain, indigestion and heartburn, abdominal pain, nausea, abdominal bloating and distention, bowel function problems (diarrhea, constipation, or both), and pain involving the rectum and anus.

Have you noticed that you tend to have distressing digestive symptoms related to poor eating, stress, or emotional distress?

Musculoskeletal (Rheumatologic) System

This system includes the muscles, soft tissues, and joints. Up to thirty percent of the population suffers from pain felt in many locations of the body. These people hurt in their muscles and joints. Doctors refer to this as chronic, widespread pain. Twenty percent of the population suffers with more localized pain, in which the pain is focused in certain bodily areas, such as the head, neck, back, or specific muscles or joints. Doctors call this *localized* or *regional pain*.

Compounding their pain problem is the fact that most people do not exercise regularly. Therefore, they are not in good condition and can have musculoskeletal pain after minimal activities. A vicious cycle sets in: exercise leads to pain, which leads to inactivity, which leads to more pain. The problem worsens with age as frailty evolves.

Are you ever consciously aware of having muscle, joint, and/or back pain associated with stress or emotional distress?

Urologic and Genital Systems

Because the urogenital systems are located in the pelvis along with the lower gastrointestinal tract (colon and rectum), it is common for symptoms from all of these systems to overlap and coexist, thereby confounding medical diagnosis. Symptoms include lower abdominal/pelvic pain and discomfort associated with altered bowel function (diarrhea, constipation, or both), frequent and/or painful urination, menstrual symptoms, prostate pain or discomfort, pelvic and genital pain, and low sexual interest or sexual dysfunction.

If you're a guy and stressed by being in a public bathroom, do you have a bashful kidney?

Autonomic (Nervous) System (ANS)

The autonomic nervous system is the part of the nervous system that automatically controls breathing, heart rate, blood pressure, sweating, and digestive function. Autonomic symptoms include shortness of breath, dizziness, fainting, rapid or slow heart rate, irregular heartbeats (palpitations), flushing, sweating, and nausea.

Do you ever notice that you are a little dizzy and that your heart races when you are stressed?

Psychological/Emotional Medically Unexplained Symptoms?

These symptoms involve the mind/brain and include thoughts ("I'm a failure"; "Nothing will get better"), beliefs, emotions, and feelings. Symptoms include feeling tense, nervous, jittery, anxious, depressed, or hopeless. Others include having difficulty concentrating or experiencing intrusive, obsessive thoughts. Compulsive/addictive behaviors are also symptoms. They may involve tobacco use, alcohol, food, sex, gambling, Internet use, and shopping. Yes, shopping! To quote Ernest Becker from his book, *The Denial of Death*,

"Modern man is drinking and drugging himself out of awareness, or he spends the time shopping, which is the same thing."

Through the *miracle* of medicalization, these symptoms often demand treatment. The ironic phrase *retail therapy* was first used in the *Chicago Tribune* on Christmas Eve, 1986. Now, it is compulsive shopping on the Internet that receives the therapist's attention. Whatever the sales approach, Ernest Becker's quote is still on the money.

Both Medically Explained and Unexplained Symptoms?

Symptoms of a medically explained disease can co-occur with medically unexplained symptoms. For example, one study found fibromyalgia to also be present in one in four patients with rheumatoid arthritis or osteoarthritis. Another example is the co-occurrence of irritable bowel syndrome with inflammatory bowel disease (ulcerative colitis or Crohn's disease) 10 to 20 percent of the time.

It is very common for symptoms to be only partially medically explained by a disease. They are, paradoxically, symptoms that are both medically explained and unexplained. For instance, symptoms may be disproportionately severe relative to the severity of the disease. One example is the person with severe heartburn caused by gastroesophageal reflux disease (GERD) who is found to have only mild acid injury inflammation (esophagitis) on endoscopic examination of the esophagus. Another example is an individual with severe abdominal pain who is found to have only a tiny ulcer. Another is a person who describes severe joint pain when the x-ray only shows mild arthritis.

Consequently, attention and treatment directed to the medically explained symptoms are either less effective than expected or ineffective. The heartburn of GERD fails to respond to powerful acid reducing therapy. The ulcer pain doesn't resolve with strong ulcer medication. The joint pain persists despite treatment.

SYMPTOMS: HERE TODAY, GONE TOMORROW?

Medically unexplained symptoms are pervasive. Many of them appear and disappear randomly and are generally not associated with any specific medical disorder. Most people pay little mind to them. Their benign nature is attested to in the doctors' medical bromide: "Take two aspirin and call me in the morning." On this point, Dr. Lewis Thomas concurs. In *The Lives of a Cell*, he states:

"The great secret, known to internists and learned early in the marriage by internists' wives, but still hidden from the general public, is that most things get better by themselves. Most things, in fact, are better by morning."

There are exceptions.

SYMPTOMS: HERE TODAY, HERE TOMORROW?

You may be reading this book because you have symptoms that are not "better by morning" or that recur so frequently that you're often not well. The constancy of recurring symptoms begins to dominate your life. You find yourself rearranging your schedule to accommodate your pain. You stop making social plans to avoid the embarrassment of your symptoms. You become isolated, frustrated, and overwhelmed. One day, you come to believe that something is really wrong and that you are no longer in control of your life. Your symptoms are in charge.

It's three A.M.

It's late, but not too late to do something about the way you feel. It's time to check out your symptoms and get relief from them once and for all. You make an appointment to see your doctor.

LINK

In the next chapter, you go to your appointment. A nurse sticks her head into the waiting room:

"The doctor will see you now."

CHAPTER 4

Symptoms Lead Us
to Doctors and Caregivers

QUESTIONS

When should I see a doctor about my symptoms?

Are they likely to be serious and can I expect to be treated and cured of them?

QUOTE

"Symptoms account for more than half of all outpatient encounters..."

Medical Clinics of North America
KURT KROENKE, M.D.
Professor of Medicine, Indiana University School of Medicine

ABOUT THE QUOTE

Kurt Kroenke, M.D., is one of the world's leading authorities in the research and management of symptoms. He is professor of medicine in the Division of General Internal Medicine and Geriatrics, Indiana University School of Medicine and a research scientist with the Regenstrief Institute. His research shows that although all people are symptomatic sometimes, seventy-five percent of them do not seek help. The twenty-five percent who do seek help account for more than one-half of all outpatient encounters. This involves nearly 400 million doctor visits per year. Among the symptomatic who seek help, approximately one-half complain of pain symptoms (headache, chest pain, abdominal pain, back pain, or joint pain), one-fourth have respiratory symptoms (mainly cough, sore throat, runny nose, and other upper respiratory symptoms related to self-limited viral infections), and one-fourth describe non-pain, non-respiratory symptoms (such as dizziness, fatigue, and heart palpitations). Most of the time, these symptoms resolve spontaneously or respond to treatment. However, about twenty-five percent of the time, they persist and recur.

In the *Medical Clinics of North America*, Drs. Kroenke and J.G. Rosmalen confirm that:

"Half of all outpatient encounters are precipitated by physical complaints, of which one-third to one-half are medically unexplained symptoms, and 20 to 25 percent are chronic or recurrent."

Many patients suffer from one or more discrete symptoms. The authors confirm that individual symptoms and somatic syndromes are associated with "impaired quality of life, increased health care use, and diminished patient and provider satisfaction."

CASE PRESENTATION:
THE DOCTOR/AUTHOR IS HERE AGAIN

I'm back to tell you about another symptom I had. I asked my wife,

"Why am I tired so much of the time?"

I felt fatigued more than I thought I should. I was fifty-nine and had just stopped making hospital rounds and taking night and weekend calls. I thought the symptom was related to too many years of hard work and stress. As an adult, I had seen doctors only about the back problems I described in Chapter 2. I had no pain. I had no other worrisome symptoms. I didn't even have a personal physician. I had no family history of heart disease. I wasn't diabetic, and my lipids (cholesterol levels) predicted low risk for me. But I finally paid attention to a remarkably subtle whisper from within,

Get your heart checked out.

I was invincible. That's what we all learned in our medical training at Vanderbilt University Hospitals, where for two years I was on call every other night, frequently with no sleep (doctors in training now have limitations on the amount of time they spend in the hospital; this protects them, and their patients). I understood that professional caregivers had to be willing to give themselves away. I had certainly been there, done that. I was still doing that. Then the doctor said,

"You have a fifty percent chance of having a flow-limiting stenosis."

I was stunned: I not only had coronary artery disease, but I also had a fifty percent chance of having a life-threatening narrowing of one or more of the main arteries to my heart! I went to see Dr. John Rumberger, a pioneering preventative cardiologist in Columbus, who took my blood pressure and ran blood tests. Then he ran me through an EBCT body scan, an electron beam CT scan of my heart, circulatory system, and body, which shows whether the arteries of the heart and circulation system have abnormal calcium in the walls. The more calcium the scan detects in the artery walls, the greater the chance there is of having a heart attack. My blood pressure was mildly elevated at times, my blood lipids should have been better, and as was noted on the scan, I had too much fat in my abdomen. He said I probably had a form of metabolic syndrome. I was very familiar with metabolic syndrome and depression, either of which could be life threatening. I believed I had both. My inner voice spoke.

You can forget what they taught you in medical school at The Ohio State University and Vanderbilt University Hospitals, because you aren't invincible after all.

With anxiety—actually fear—I called my friend and colleague, Dr. David Bichsel, an excellent cardiologist in Columbus who worked at my hospital. He told me I had mild coronary artery disease and that I should have a nuclear cardiac stress test to be on the safe side, even though I never had chest pain during strenuous exercise. I had always been the doctor. Now I became the patient. I thought to myself,

You've flunked the stress test and you're a patient!

I also recalled the words of one of my favorite teachers at Vanderbilt. Dr. Clifton Meador was fond of reminding his students,

"The only safe way to go into a hospital is to have a white coat on."

Dr. Bichsel recommended cardiac catheterization, which confirmed Dr. Rumberger's concern that there was a tight narrowing in my right coronary artery, the main artery supplying blood to my heart. I have coronary artery disease and now have a coronary stent in my heart.

I am okay now. I eat healthily and exercise. I take medication and supplements to improve my cholesterol levels. My fatigue has resolved. I don't think I am depressed anymore. Thanks to the care of John and Dave, I intend never to have a heart attack. But I get it. My prognosis is up to me. Three years later, particularly after observing how Tom has improved his health in retirement and shortly after completing the first draft of this book with him, I retired from medicine and gastroenterology.

SECOND CASE PRESENTATION

"What brings you to see me?" the doctor asks.

The patient says, "It is my pain. It's been going on for a long time, probably several years, and it's getting worse. I've been putting up with it too long, and I'm worried that it's serious. It's really beginning to interfere with my life. I get cramps in my lower abdomen. I'm usually constipated, but when the pain comes, I have diarrhea. The pain goes away once I stop going. Things are worse if I'm stressed or upset. I haven't seen any blood in my bowel movements, and my appetite is all right. I haven't lost weight. In fact, it keeps going up. And the pain isn't just in my abdomen. I hurt all over. It's as if I have arthritis everywhere. There's no swelling of my joints. I don't think I have a fever. But the pain is really upsetting. I don't have much energy, and I have a lot of trouble sleeping."

All of the medical tests are normal.

THE MOST COMMON SYMPTOM: PAIN

The two case studies are symptomatically revealing. The most common symptom that people have is pain. While the fatigue described in the first presentation was a medically explained symptom, the chronic pain felt by the patient in the second presentation was not.

Most chronic pain is medically unexplained.

Pain complaints account for over one-half of all outpatient visits for symptoms. Doctors are under great pressure to help patients manage pain. The Joint Commission for Accreditation of Healthcare Organizations and the Veterans Administration require routine measurement of pain (*the fifth vital sign*—the other four being heart rate, respiratory rate, blood pressure, and temperature). Chronic pain is among the leading causes of both temporary and permanent work disability. Chronic pain often leads to expensive, uncomfortable, and sometimes risky medical tests and can result in unneeded surgery. It is the primary reason that people use complementary and alternative medicine. Despite all this, true multidisciplinary pain clinics are neither widely available nor regularly reimbursed by insurance providers and other health care payers. Moreover, pharmaceutical treatment is not always a viable option. Doctors avoid prescribing narcotics for chronic pain that is not associated with cancer. Their reluctance is a twofold concern. They must comply with regulatory restrictions. They must protect patients from developing dependency or addiction. Therefore, pain management by prescription has limitations. Pain itself does not. It persists as the most common symptom of the symptomatic.

WHY PEOPLE WITH SYMPTOMS DECIDE TO SEE THE DOCTOR

There are several reasons people decide they need help from a medical professional regarding their symptoms:

→ **Severity:** "This pain is really bad."
→ **Chronicity:** "I've had these headaches for too long now."
→ **Progression:** "I've been tired for a while, but it's getting worse."
→ **Concerns and expectations:** "Is this pain harmless and going to go away, or is it something serious that might be life-threatening?"
→ **Associated psychological factors (e.g., depression and/or anxiety):** "The pain is depressing me." or "These symptoms are making me nervous."

Whatever the reason for deciding to see the doctor, the patient and his/her physician must confront the Symptoms Iceberg.

THE SYMPTOMS ICEBERG HAS CHANGED

Dr. Kroenke says:

"Physical symptoms presenting in the clinic represent only the tip of the iceberg, since less than one-fourth of symptomatic patients in the community come to the clinic for their symptoms."

We introduced the Symptoms Iceberg in Chapter 1. It represents all of the symptoms that people could possibly experience. But, according to modern medical science, its mass is different than it once was. Over the past one hundred years, it has grown.

Now the iceberg is larger. More people have more symptoms. Picture the iceberg floating higher in the water, so that more of the iceberg is visible. The tip is larger, showing that people are more likely than ever to see the doctor about symptoms. Studies show that approximately twenty-five percent of symptomatic people decide to consult with one or more doctors. Dr. Edward Shorter, who holds the Hannah Chair in the History of Medicine at the University of Toronto, has researched and written extensively about medically unexplained symptoms. He has confirmed that:

People are becoming increasingly likely to seek professional help for their symptoms.

This observation is based upon epidemiological studies of ambulatory practice, surveys of public attitudes, and historical examination of medical practice. People are increasingly aware of, bothered, and disabled by pain, symptoms, and illness, which in the past were not considered important or worthy enough to need medical attention. There are many reasons for this phenomenon, and we refer the reader to Dr. Shorter's book, *Doctors and Their Patients*, for his analysis. We have also introduced to you the concept of medicalization. Harvard doctors Arthur Barsky and Jonathan Borus observe that people's tolerance of symptoms has decreased, thus contributing to "progressive medicalization of physical distress in which uncomfortable bodily states and isolated symptoms are classified as diseases." Consider reviewing the process of medicalization that we discussed in the first chapter.

HOW DOCTORS SEE SYMPTOMS

In medicine, symptoms are either: 1) explained by the medical diagnosis of a specific disease, or 2) not so clearly explained. Both patient and doctor usually understand medically explained symptoms, but neither understands medically unexplained symptoms, and this is the basis for trouble with a capital T. Here's why.

MEDICALLY EXPLAINED SYMPTOMS (A LINEAR PROCESS)

When seen clearly, symptoms may lead both the patient and doctor to a diagnosis, which is confirmed by medical testing. For example, shortness of breath, chest pain, and fever lead to a diagnosis of bacterial pneumonia on chest x-ray. Burning on urination and passage of blood in the urine lead to the diagnosis of a bacterial urinary tract infection based on abnormal urinalysis and urine culture. With the diagnosis confirmed, there is clear sailing for both patients and doctors. From symptoms to diagnosis, the process of evaluation is linear: A (the symptoms) are caused by B (the specific diagnosis). Medical tests for A confirm B. Treatment of B with antibiotics cures and relieves A.

Patients and doctors understand.

MEDICALLY UNEXPLAINED SYMPTOMS (A NON-LINEAR COMPLEX PROCESS)

Most of the time, symptoms are not readily explainable by medical diagnosis because medical evaluation and testing fail to show a cause. The March 1989 issue of *The American Journal of Medicine* has an article entitled, "Common Symptoms in Ambulatory Care: Incidence, Evaluation, Therapy, and Outcome," that has been referenced thousands of times. In it, Dr. Kroenke and his colleague, A.D. Mangelsdorff, report their findings on symptoms diagnosis. From their research, they confirm that during the evaluation of the fourteen most common symptoms seen in primary care practice, doctors found a definite organic cause only sixteen percent of the time. Their findings reinforce what has become an enormously difficult problem for doctors.

Trying to explain the unexplainable to patients usually leads to misunderstanding.

The doctor makes a syndrome diagnosis because medical tests fail to show a cause for the symptoms. They are medically unexplainable. A colonoscopy fails to explain the symptoms of abdominal pain and bowel problems. Therefore, the doctor diagnoses irritable bowel syndrome (IBS), which is a symptom-based diagnosis. Tests for arthritis and other medical disorders do not explain symptoms of hurting all over, which are associated with fatigue. Therefore, the doctor diagnoses fibromyalgia syndrome (FMS), which is another symptom-based diagnosis. This phenomenon is the subject of the next chapter.

When symptoms are unexplainable, the diagnostic directional course is unclear, difficult, and treacherous.

Visualize how hard it is to see the Symptoms Iceberg because it is dark and shrouded in fog. This is what it is like for doctor and patient. Neither can see clearly what is behind or beneath the observable symptoms. Life becomes more difficult than it already is because nothing is clear. For the doctor, the concept of the unexplainable doesn't fit. The concept isn't linear. While it's true that A (the symptoms) lead to B (the diagnosis), the diagnostic labels used above refer to vague and strange diseases that lack medical confirmation. The doctor makes the diagnosis based upon his or her recognition, description, and collection of symptoms (A). Furthermore, treatment commonly doesn't relieve them. Picture that now there is darkness and fog around the iceberg. No one can see clearly how big it is, let alone what lies beneath the surface.

BOTH MEDICALLY EXPLAINED
AND UNEXPLAINED SYMPTOMS

As you learned in Chapter 3, it is also common for symptoms to be only partially medically explained by a disease; that is, they are both medically explained and unexplained. Sometimes, too, symptoms are stronger than would be expected based upon evaluation of the severity of the disease. Attention and treatment directed to the medically explained symptoms are either less effective than expected or ineffective. This discordance can lead to potentially dangerous testing and treatment. You can imagine how frustrating this is for both doctor and patient. More than you imagine, you may have been on the receiving end of treatment that doesn't work. Hoping for clear sailing, your symptoms remain unexplained.

You want a name put to what you are experiencing. You want an explanation!

But the name comes at a cost.

LINK

In the next chapter, we chip away at the Symptoms Iceberg and describe how doctors put labels on the unexplainable and diagnose syndromes from symptoms.

CHAPTER 5

We Receive a Syndrome Diagnosis

QUESTIONS

What is a symptom syndrome known as a "functional somatic syndrome"?

How is it diagnosed, and can it be cured?

QUOTE

*"What's in a name? That which we call a rose
by any other name would smell as sweet."*

Romeo and Juliet (II, ii, 1-2)
WILLIAM SHAKESPEARE

ABOUT THE QUOTE

Shakespeare's dramas observe and pierce cultural convention. In the quote above, Juliet, by analogy, gets behind the status labeling of family names to capture Romeo's essence. What is in a name? Jerome Groopman, M.D., is a Harvard professor of medicine. In "Hurting All Over," an article published in the November 13, 2000 issue of *The New Yorker*, he writes,

"Of all the words a doctor uses, the name he gives the illness has the greatest weight."

He is correct when he goes on to say that the name, the diagnosis, becomes the basis for all later discussion and dialogue between not only patient and doctor, but also between doctor and doctor and between patient and patient. The name can be used to explain the illness to others as well as to the patient. The name labels the patient. Like Velcro, it sticks to the one diagnosed, especially if the name given is syndrome.

Merriam-Webster Online defines the word *syndrome* as:

1. a group of signs and symptoms that occur together and characterize a particular abnormality or condition;
2. a set of concurrent things (as emotions or actions) that usually form an identifiable pattern.

When medically unexplained symptoms, a set of emotions, and/or a set of actions (behaviors) occur together, doctors group them and diagnose one or more symptom syndromes. In this book, the words *syndrome* and *disorder* will mean the same thing.

What is the consequence of this?

In many respects, the name of the illness becomes part of the identity of the patient.

The words of a symptom syndrome diagnosis often paint patients into a corner, which results in misunderstanding and frustration for both patients and doctors, as the following case study demonstrates.

CASE PRESENTATION

M. A. is a forty-five-year-old teacher who decided to consult with WBS because of generalized abdominal pain and bloating associated with alternating diarrhea and constipation. Her primary care physician told her that she had irritable bowel syndrome. She didn't know what it was or what to do about it, and the medication her doctor prescribed didn't work. Their ten minutes together had not permitted exploration of all the other symptoms that she had. So she ended up consulting with three other specialists:

A RHEUMATOLOGIST diagnosed fibromyalgia syndrome because of widespread pain associated with fatigue.

Her GYNECOLOGIST diagnosed chronic pelvic pain syndrome.

The UROLOGIST diagnosed irritable bladder syndrome because of painful and frequent urination.

She returned to her primary care physician because medical treatments weren't working. The doctor advised her to return to specialists. Until she saw WBS, none of the other doctors had suggested that there might be some relationship between her various symptoms and diagnoses, let alone suggested that there could be an underlying cause. Two did suggest she might be depressed. After each visit, she had the impression that the doctor was irritated and frustrated with her. She felt that they all suspected that she was depressed. She wondered if she was depressed because of the pain.

DOCTORS CLASSIFY MEDICALLY UNEXPLAINED SYMPTOMS

Dr. Kurt Kroenke classifies medically unexplained symptoms into five general categories:

1. Partially explained by a medical disorder;
2. Symptom only diagnosis;
3. Functional somatic syndrome;
4. Primary psychiatric disorder (depression and anxiety); and
5. Somatoform disorder.

We consider Dr. Kroenke's classification of medically unexplained symptoms to be very helpful, so let's look at it in detail.

1. Partially Explained by a Medical Disorder

In this situation, the symptoms are not responding to standard treatment and/or are not proportionate to the medical severity of the disorder. Heartburn and indigestion are described as severe, but they fail to respond to drugs, even though an endoscopic exam reveals no inflammation or abnormality. Another example is chest pain in a patient who has mild coronary artery disease, which is related more to stress than findings on cardiac stress testing. A third is the severe pain of mild rheumatoid arthritis that does not respond to powerful anti-arthritic therapy.

2. Symptom Only Diagnosis

Symptoms are simply described as a diagnosis, without an attempt to propose a cause for them. Examples here include diagnosis of low back pain, dyspepsia, abdominal pain, and dizziness. The criteria for diagnosis are vague, which leads to much variation in diagnostic testing and treatment.

3. Functional Somatic Syndrome

Along with other experts, Harvard physicians Arthur Barsky and Jonathan Borus explain in the *Annals of Internal Medicine* that:

"Every medical specialty has an approach to the recognition and diagnosis of medically unexplained symptoms that falls within its area of expertise."

Collections of medically unexplained symptoms are given a diagnostic name.

In medical specialties, these symptom syndromes are called *functional somatic syndromes*, the most common of which are listed below.

GASTROENTEROLOGY: irritable bowel syndrome (and over thirty other syndromes)

RHEUMATOLOGY: fibromyalgia syndrome

CARDIOLOGY: non-cardiac chest pain; mitral valve prolapse

PULMONOLOGY (RESPIRATORY MEDICINE): hyperventilation syndrome; vocal cord dysfunction

GYNECOLOGY: premenstrual syndrome; chronic pelvic pain syndrome

INFECTIOUS DISEASE: chronic fatigue syndrome

NEUROLOGY: chronic headaches

OTOLARYNGOLOGY (EAR, NOSE AND THROAT): dizziness; globus; temporomandibular joint disorder (TMJD); facial pain disorder; vocal cord dysfunction

DENTISTRY: facial pain disorder; temporomandibular joint disorder

ALLERGY: multiple chemical sensitivity (MCS) / idiopathic environmental intolerance (IEI); multiple drug intolerance syndrome

ORTHOPEDIC SURGERY: chronic back pain

UROLOGY: painful bladder syndrome (interstitial cystitis); painful prostate syndrome (chronic prostatitis)

SURGERY: chronic functional abdominal pain syndrome

ALL SPECIALTIES: multiple chemical sensitivity (MCS)/idiopathic environmental intolerance (IEI); multiple drug intolerance syndrome

This book is about asking the right questions to get the right answers. Writing in the British medical journal *The Lancet*, doctors involved with research of medically unexplained symptoms ask a question in the title of the article:

"Functional somatic syndromes: one or many?"

Keep this important question in mind as you read on.

4. Primary Psychiatric Disorder

There are hundreds of psychiatric disorders described in the *Diagnostic and Statistical Manual of Mental Disorders, Fourth Edition, Text Revi-*

sion (DSM-IV-TR). Several are associated with otherwise medically unexplained symptoms. The two most common psychiatric syndromes are depression and anxiety. Two rare disorders are factitious disorder and malingering.

Depression and/or Anxiety

In current medical practice, doctors consider undiagnosed depression and/or anxiety to be at least associated with medically unexplained symptoms, if not the most common causes of them. We have *lumped* depression with anxiety here because the reality in medicine is that it can be very difficult to distinguish one from the other.

Doctors address medical symptoms without identified pathology and their relationship to psychiatric disorders in the 1 May, 2001 supplement issue of the *Annals of Internal Medicine*, as referred to in Chapter 3. The association of medically unexplained physical symptoms with depression and the frequent diagnosis of depression as causative are extremely important observations that will be explored in depth in the next chapter.

While other medically unexplained symptoms can be associated with depression, the most common are listed as follows:

→ Fatigue;
→ Energy (low);
→ Pain (e.g., headache, neck and back, abdomen);
→ Weight change (loss or gain);
→ Appetite change (loss or gain); and
→ Libido (loss).

Medically unexplained symptoms associated with anxiety are:

→ Fatigue;
→ Sleep difficulties;
→ Irritability and difficulty concentrating;
→ Dizziness or lightheadedness;
→ Hot flashes or chills;
→ Sweating;
→ Trembling or shaking;
→ Muscle tension;
→ Choking feeling or tightness in the throat;
→ Dry mouth;
→ Tingling or numbness in the hands or feet;
→ Chest pressure or chest pain;

→ Abdominal pain;
→ Pounding heart and/or racing pulse;
→ Shortness of breath;
→ Nausea;
→ Extreme fear of losing control, doing something embarrassing, going crazy, or dying; and
→ Sense of feeling unreal or being in a dreamlike state.

The three most common anxiety syndromes are generalized anxiety disorder, panic disorder, and specific phobias.

Generalized Anxiety Disorder (GAD)

GAD is ongoing worry or fear that isn't related to a particular event or situation, or is out of proportion to what would be expected. An example would be constantly worrying about a child who is perfectly healthy. Any symptoms listed above can occur, but typically include muscle tension, trembling, shortness of breath, fast heartbeat, dry mouth, dizziness, nausea, irritability, loss of sleep, and lack of concentration.

Panic Disorder

Repeated episodes of extreme anxiety-associated symptoms are called *panic attacks*. The person does not know what triggers the attack. The attacks last from five to thirty minutes and may include any of the symptoms listed. An example of a panic attack is the sudden onset of dizziness, a racing and pounding heart, fear of losing control, and chest pain occurring for no apparent reason. Panic attacks can lead to phobias.

Phobia

A phobia is an extreme, unreasonable fear in response to something specific. Examples include anxiety about being in places where it is difficult or embarrassing to escape (agoraphobia) and being in a small and confined place (claustrophobia).

Factitious Disorder

Patients diagnosed with factitious disorder intentionally manifest disease. Their sole purpose in assuming the sick role rests in an inner need to be seen as ill or injured rather than a need to achieve an external benefit, such as financial gain. An extreme example of factitious disorder is the Munchausen syndrome, in which the patient deliberately produces or exaggerates physical symptoms in various ways, such as lying about or faking symptoms, causing self-injury, or altering diagnostic tests. The self-induction of disease is often not recognized at first. Factitious disorder patients who feign a psychiatric illness can be even harder to recognize.

Malingering

Malingering is feigning or grossly exaggerating physical or emotional/psychological symptoms. In contrast, patients with medically unexplained symptoms do not feign or intentionally produce their symptoms.

5. Somatoform Disorder

These are psychiatric diagnoses in which the patient is preoccupied with physical symptoms including pain, the most common symptom experience. Medical tests fail to show a specific physical cause. Depression and anxiety are not present. There is no substance abuse. Patients diagnosed with somatoform disorder have typically presented different symptoms for several years.

The list below describes the medically unexplained symptoms that commonly lead to a psychiatric somatoform syndrome diagnosis:

→ Main concern and worry about symptoms: SOMATIZATION;
→ Loss of function (e.g., weakness in an extremity): CONVERSION;
→ Predominant symptom is pain: PAIN DISORDER;
→ Main concern and worry about disease: HYPOCHONDRIASIS;
→ Dislike of body parts: BODY DYSMORPHIC DISORDER.

COMORBIDITY: THE SOMEWHAT SCARY MEDICAL TERM THAT REFERS TO THE *ASSOCIATION* AND COEXISTENCE OF MEDICALLY UNEXPLAINED SYMPTOM SYNDROMES

In medicine and psychiatry, the term *comorbidity* refers to the presence of one or more disorders or diseases in addition to a primary disorder or disease. In "Review of the Evidence for Overlap among Unexplained Clinical Conditions," published in the prominent medical journal *Annals of Internal Medicine*, two doctors reviewed fifty-three studies that examined the association/coexistence of two or more syndromes in groups of patients. They found overlapping occurrences of the following symptom syndromes:

→ 35 to 70 percent for fibromyalgia syndrome and chronic fatigue syndrome;

→ 32 to 80 percent for fibromyalgia syndrome and irritable bowel syndrome;

→ 58 to 92 percent for chronic fatigue syndrome and irritable bowel syndrome;

→ 33 to 55 percent for fibromyalgia syndrome and multiple chemical sensitivity;

→ 30 to 67 percent for chronic fatigue syndrome and multiple chemical sensitivity.

Recall the question asked by the British physicians in *The Lancet*:

"Functional somatic syndromes: one or many?"

Based upon a comprehensive review of previous studies, both groups of researchers conclude that there is substantial overlap between the individual syndromes and that the similarities between them outweigh the differences.

FEELING BAD IN MORE WAYS THAN ONE

In 2007, an important medical study was published in the *Journal of General Internal Medicine*, "Feeling Bad in More Ways than One: Comorbidity Patterns of Medically Unexplained and Psychiatric Conditions." The researchers found that the association/coexistence of the following nine conditions far exceeded chance expectations: chronic fatigue, low back pain, irritable bowel syndrome, chronic tension headache, fibromyalgia, temporomandibular joint disorder, major depression, panic attacks, and posttraumatic stress disorder.

These experts found that:

"These results [the common concurrence of medically unexplained and psychiatric conditions] support theories suggesting that medically unexplained conditions share a common etiology."

These findings and conclusion deserve everybody's close attention. However, you have seen how time constraints and other problems in the medical realm dictate little chance for in-depth scrutiny and evaluation.

MEDICAL MELTDOWN

The patient and doctor have very little time to spend with one another (the reasons for this are the topic of another discussion).

The average doctor visit lasts for less than ten minutes!

During this incredibly short time, the doctor stares up at the giant Symptoms Iceberg and must first distinguish medically explainable symptoms from those that are medically unexplainable. The doctor also knows that the symptoms may be both medically explainable and medically unexplainable. If they are medically explainable, the patient and doctor share an understanding of the medical problem. When the symptoms are not medically explainable or are both, the doctor and the patient share frustration. To alleviate frustration, the doctor tries to reduce the size of the symptoms iceberg by aggregating collections of unexplained symptoms into symptom syndromes.

This leads to a medical meltdown for everybody involved.

Here are five reasons why:

1. The "diagnostic" syndrome labels are defined and classified by specialists and subspecialists

For example, gastroenterologists diagnose abdominal pain associated with bowel dysfunction as irritable bowel syndrome. Rheumatologists diagnose widespread pain associated with fatigue as fibromyalgia. Each specialty offers and applies its own diagnostic and therapeutic approach. Furthermore, if a syndrome overlaps more than one specialty, then the label and treatment may vary considerably, depending upon the specialist diagnosing the problem. Take one example. Chronic back pain may be described as *facet syndrome* and treated with local injections by the pain specialist and/or anesthesiologist; as *subluxation* treated with manipulation by the osteopath; as *instability* treated with surgery by the orthopedic surgeon or neurosurgeon; as *depression* treated with antidepressants by the psychiatrist; or as *somatization/illness behavior* treated with cognitive behavioral therapy by the psychologist.

2. Syndromes frequently share core symptoms

For example, both fibromyalgia syndrome and chronic fatigue syndrome include the symptom of fatigue, which raises diagnostic uncertainty regarding any singular syndrome diagnosis.

3. Syndromes and other medically unexplained symptoms often coexist

Nevertheless, specialists usually disregard the significance of these coexisting symptoms and syndromes and focus attention upon the symptom and/or symptom syndrome within their area of expertise.

4. With functional symptom syndromes, there is a communications gap between patients and doctors

Patients' perceptions of their symptoms are underestimated by the doctors. Views diverge on best treatment options. Patients consider a single test that would uncover the *cause* as the most desirable one. But most patients do not *own* a doctor's *functional* diagnosis. Often they either deny being given the diagnosis or are skeptical about it being a firm or *real* diagnosis.

5. There is a strong link between medically unexplained symptoms and depression and stress

This is a very difficult matter for both patient and doctor that will be discussed in detail in the next chapter. Doctors face the dilemma of distinguishing normal human emotion and behavior from symptomatic emotions and behaviors that reflect a significant psychological dysfunction. Consequently, both doctors and patients may resort to drug therapy. As a result, there has been an enormous increase in the use of antidepressant medications. Today, ten percent of Americans are on antidepressants, and many more have taken them. Accordingly, there is an important question to ask,

For most of us, is feeling sad—or having the associated medically unexplained physical symptoms of depression—a major depression syndrome?

Allan Horwitz, dean of social and behavioral sciences at Rutgers, and Jerome Wakefield, an expert on mental illness diagnosis at New York University, have written an important book, *The Loss of Sadness: How Psychiatry Transformed Normal Sorrow into Depressive Disorder*. In the book, they warn that the apparent epidemic of depression in fact reflects the way medicine and the psychiatric profession in particular has reinterpreted and reclassified normal human sadness as largely an abnormal experience. They argue that the current approach to diagnosing depression is based upon the presence of symptoms for periods as short as two or more weeks. Only five symptoms, including such common ones as depressed mood, weight gain, insomnia, fatigue, and indecisiveness are necessary for the diagnosis of a major depressive disorder, based upon the *Diagnostic and Statistical Manual of Mental Disorders* (DSM) published by the American Psychiatric Association.

There is a potential flaw in this diagnostic approach if it fails to consider the context in which the symptoms occur.

There's a difference between the abnormal reactions of a patient with major depression syndrome and a normal reaction of sadness any of us feel as part of the human experience.

The former reflects a disconnectedness and imbalance occurring within the patient's psyche, along with possible neurotransmitter imbalance. The latter is an emotive, connective response to the reality that life is hard and sometimes sorrowful. While an experienced diagnostician would take this into account and not just base diagnosis on the symptoms, it is possible, under the current DSM classification system, that someone might not make the distinction. The expected symptoms related to upsetting life experiences—for example, the end of a relationship or loss of a job—could be the basis for the diagnosis of a depressive syndrome.

WHAT'S NORMAL?

What is disorder and what is underlying normal? As discussed in the first chapter, the medicalization and consequent diagnoses of what were once considered daily life problems and issues is one cause of the epidemic of symptoms. The doctor has no time to explain this. There is no time to probe what's behind the symptoms. There is no common language between patients and doctors to communicate what is really going on. Telling patients that the tests are normal may relieve some of them. But for many, there is the feeling that the doctor thinks this is all in the patient's head. Finally, when symptoms cannot be explained, there is no way to link them to their cause. Medical treatment is ineffective and has no cure.

WHO CARES?

When symptoms are medically unexplainable and may involve more than one syndrome, diagnostic fragmentation is inevitable. Each specialty homes in on its own area of expertise. Care is disjointed because of the number and diversity of professionals involved. There is little communication and integration. Frustration is high for everybody. Ordering tests, prescribing medication, and facilitating other medical treatment suffer from a lack of coordination. Costs run out of control.

THERE ARE LAYERS

Patients with medically unexplained symptoms often manifest symptomatically in more than one of the five symptom categories Dr. Kroenke has identified. This intensifies the doctor's evaluation dilemma. In addition to time constraints, the doctor sees only what is above the surface and only to the depth that his or her training and tools allow him or her to see. However,

People are layered.

What we mean by this is that each of us is complex and multifaceted. We are shaped genetically and multi-systemically by the familial, social, educational, and spiritual environments in which we were raised and we now function. We often present ourselves based on who we think we should be and who others expect us to be. Deep within each of us is the *who I really am*. It is hidden under the layers and difficult to detect, especially during a ten-minute consultation.

In the brief time that doctors and other caregivers have to spend with their patients and care receivers, it is impossible to explore and truly understand life's narratives, which include matters of mind/brain, body, and soul, influenced by multiple biological and environmental factors. Attempts at categorization commonly trivialize and/or worsen distress.

PAINTED INTO A SPOTLIT CORNER

All too often, the diagnosis itself stifles and replaces effective communication and education. The diagnosis of medically unexplained symptoms and syndromes is but a name. It's a label. The word or words named aloud should contribute to a patient's self-understanding and sense of inclusion in the portrait of the human family.

Instead, the label paints patients into an isolated corner—and doctors and other care givers into their own corners—where despite the spotlight, they all feel alone and misunderstood.

Dr. Kroenke says,

"Medically unexplained symptoms are a major public health problem."

What's in a name? When it's a syndrome label that leaves both patient and doctor cornered, frustrated, and further stressed, what's in it is an opportunity lost. Understanding succumbs to misunderstanding, hope and healing to no cure. Far from sweet, this is medicine's bitter pill.

SICK OF SYMPTOMS REVISITED

Recall the study described in Chapter 1, which found that,

"More than half of U.S. adults have a physical or mental condition that prevents them from working or conducting their usual duties for several days each year."

Medically unexplained symptoms and functional somatic syndromes can result in significant impairment of the quality of life. Consequent disability is a worldwide problem. A recent international study published in the *Journal of Psychosomatic Research* shows that patients in diverse cultures who had five or more explained or unexplained bodily symptoms had increased psychosocial morbidity and physical disability. Medically unexplained symptoms and functional somatic syndromes are also often associated with depression. This link is itself an important cause of quality of life deterioration and disability.

MEDICATION AND TREATMENT

Medications and treatments are available for several of the functional somatic syndromes and psychiatric syndromes. Possibly helpful in treating symptoms, they will be discussed in the next chapter and in **PART 4:** Learn How Doctors Think and How to Work with Them. For now, please keep in mind that:

Fragmentation within the medical system further contributes to the confusion and frustration as caring professionals and patients fail to appreciate and address the significance of associated syndromes.

LINK

In the next chapter, you will begin to explore the remarkable association of medically unexplained symptoms with depression and stress and discover the truth of the mind/brain – body connections.

CHAPTER 6

The Diagnosis of Depression Describes a Double Hurt

QUESTIONS

Why are so many people taking antidepressant medications?
Is there an association of depression with disease and symptoms?
Is there an association of stress with disease and symptoms?

QUOTES

"I am no better in mind than in body; both alike are sick and I suffer double hurt."

Tristia. Ex Ponto

OVID

"Pain and depression are the most common physical and psychological symptoms in primary care, respectively. Moreover, they co-occur 30% to 50% of the time and have adverse effects on quality of life, disability, and health care costs."

Journal of the American Medical Association May 27, 2009

DR. KURT KROENKE AND COLLEAGUES

"1 in 10 is taking medication to improve mood and fewer are going for talk therapy."

Archives of General Psychiatry (August, 2009)

DOCTORS MARK OLFSON AND STEVEN MARCUS

ABOUT THE QUOTES

The remarkable quotation from Ovid reflects an ancient understanding of the reciprocal relationship of the mind/brain with the body. Each affects the other. The quote from Dr. Kroenke reinforces both how common medically unexplained physical symptoms and depression are and how often they occur together. As Dr. Kroenke also indicates, they impair quality of life, contribute to disability, and increase health care costs. The third quote refers to findings in an important medical study reported in the August 2009 issue of the *Archives of General Psychiatry*. Use of antidepressant drugs in the United States doubled between 1996 and 2005.

Ten percent of people age six or older are taking antidepressant drugs.

When you are sick and in pain, you suffer double hurt, because both mind/brain and body are involved. For many reasons, this ancient sense of an integrated self has become lost on most people, including doctors. It has been displaced by modern Western science, which views the mind/brain as separate from the body. This shift has profoundly affected how medicine thinks about health and disease.

For centuries, culturally diverse healing traditions shared a holistic vantage point on the unity of mind, body, and universe. Native American, Western Hippocratic, Indian Ayurvedic, and Chinese medical healers characterized health as the harmony and balance of this unity. Illness and disease reflected a loss of this balance. In his book, *Timeless Healing*, Harvard's Herbert Benson, M.D., writes:

"A review of ancient history shows that we are returning to original beliefs that the mind and body cannot be separated."

CASE PRESENTATION

N. L. is a thirty-eight-year-old married housewife and supermarket cashier who consulted me with a one-year history of generalized abdominal pain and bloating, alternating constipation and diarrhea, and an unexplained twenty-five-pound weight gain. She felt fatigued and suffered from generalized aches and pains. She had seen four other doctors and received diagnoses of irritable bowel syndrome, fibromyalgia syndrome, and chronic fatigue syndrome. One doctor suggested that she was depressed and prescribed an antidepressant drug for her.

I asked her four important questions:

1. "What is going on in your life now and how are you feeling about it?"

2. "What do you think is wrong with you?"
3. "What are you worried might be wrong with you?"
4. "What is your self-care plan?"

She responded that she was under a lot of stress, particularly because she was so sick. She did not understand her diagnoses. She was worried that she had cancer or some other serious disease. She was offended that one of the doctors thought she was depressed, and she said that *if* she really were depressed, then it was because of the symptoms. She reluctantly took the antidepressant medication, but it had not been particularly helpful. She couldn't understand what self-care had to do with her problems. She couldn't see any connection.

SPLITTING MIND AND BODY

Dr. Shelley E. Taylor is a health psychologist at UCLA. In her textbook, *Health Psychology*, she indicates that most evidence suggests that ancient people considered the mind and body as a unit. Over time, the perspective of caregivers shifted. With the Renaissance came new understandings of the human body, health, and disease. Scientific discovery and new technology, particularly the microscope, spurred the advances. Medicine turned increasingly to scientific investigation of the body, rather than the mind, as the basis for medical progress. Western scientific thought began to displace the ancients' holistic view. The mind was now separate from the body. No longer about mind/body imbalance, disease was a mechanical failure of body parts that needed to be repaired.

Gradually, Western medicine fixated on a repair shop mindset.

With the shift, physicians explored bodily illness and disease from a scientific, linear, and constricted perspective. Recall that the linear concept of cause and effect regarding medically explained symptoms is that: symptoms (A) are caused by the disease (B). All types of sophisticated diagnostic testing, drug therapy, and surgical treatment work well when things are linear and the symptoms (A) are medically explained and caused by the disease (B).

But this linear model of understanding fails completely when it comes to medically unexplained symptoms—both psychological/emotional and physical—and, most notably, those that are associated with depression and stress.

When things are not linear and the symptoms (A) lead to a mysterious symptom-based diagnosis (B), the scientific method and modern medical model of treatment are less the tools of cure than broken mechanisms themselves.

They can neither imagine what is behind the symptoms nor integrate them into a holistic system of cause and effect.

SPLITTING YOU

Up to this point, we have focused upon how symptoms are arbitrarily split into categories, based upon whether they are either psychological/ emotional (e.g. depression, anxiety) or physical (e.g. pain, bowel disturbance, fatigue). Physical symptoms are further split apart from the whole person. As described in Chapter 3, they can be categorized as constitutional/vital, such as fatigue and insomnia, or they can be attributed to the gastrointestinal, musculoskeletal, urologic, or autonomic systems. Splitting symptoms into these categories not only doesn't work, it makes matters worse. Accordingly, these words attributed to Cicero hit home:

"In a disordered mind, as in a disordered body, soundness of health is impossible."

The medical world views you from a fragmented perspective. No wonder your symptoms may cause you to see yourself as fragmented and broken. In the healing arts, we have forgotten where we came from. Consequently, the holistic big picture regarding symptoms and health is blurry.

Mind/brain and body suffer a double hurt.

But too few raise the question of what this means. However, by asking the right questions, people can find the right answers for the underlying causes of what ails them. By asking, they reiterate the age-old inquiry into the integral association of health with the relationships of body, mind, spirit, and the physical and social world around us (the environment). So we ask you now to read again the three questions that open this chapter.

The *association* of depression and stress with disease and symptoms is the key that will open the door to self-understanding and allow you to see what your symptoms have to say regarding what being human and healthy is all about.

Take a closer look at the depression, symptoms, and disease association.

DEPRESSION AND DISEASE/SYMPTOMS

You now know how common depression is.

The Depression Epidemic

Doctors and other care-giving professionals see an epidemic of depression, but the big picture of depression is much less clear for both patients and professionals. Depression can be major, minor (episodic and less severe), and *dysthymic* (chronic low-grade depression). In any given one-year period, the National Institute of Mental Health reports that 9.5 percent of the population—approximately 20.9 million American adults—suffers from a depressive illness. Furthermore, one out of four will do so at some time in life. Children and adolescents are increasingly affected, and the problem is worldwide. The World Health Organization reports that depression is the leading cause of disability and the fourth leading cause of disease worldwide.

There is no question that major depression can be a significant cause of debilitating, life-threatening illness, which requires medical care and treatment. Depression is common, chronic, and costly.

Reporting in the *Journal of the American Medical Association* in 2003, researchers find that employers lose an estimated $44 billion every year due to workers with clinical depression.

The Depression—Disease Link

Science has confirmed a powerful association between depression and serious medical conditions, including every element of metabolic syndrome (excess weight/obesity, high blood pressure, cholesterol abnormalities, elevated blood sugar and diabetes, and fatty liver.) Depression increases the risk of heart disease in healthy persons and increases the risk of dying in those who have had heart attacks. Depression is even associated with osteoporosis. In the *Medical Clinics of North America*, Dr. R.O. Gans of the University Medical Center, Groningen, Netherlands has a 2006 article entitled, "The Metabolic Syndrome, Depression, and Cardiovascular Disease: Interrelated Conditions that Share Pathophysiologic Mechanisms." In it, he argues for "a more integrative approach to patients in general that surpass[es] the current disease-centered services such as endocrinology, psychiatry, and cardiology."

In a 2008 report published in *General Hospital Psychiatry*, doctors and researchers (including Indiana University's Dr. Kurt Kroenke) associated with the Division of Adult and Community Health, Centers for Disease Control and Prevention, Atlanta, GA conclude:

"The associations between depression, anxiety, obesity, and unhealthy behaviors among U.S. adults suggest the need for a multidimensional and integrative approach to health care."

Let's explore these links further.

The Depression—Symptoms Link

Dr. Kroenke says that in the current medical model, one out of every five patients seen in a primary care medical practice comes in with symptoms associated with depression. Diagnosis is easier when classical psychological/emotional symptoms of depression are present, like low mood, loss of interest in the pleasures of life, poor concentration, anxiety, and feelings of helplessness, hopelessness, or worthlessness.

However, the reality is that symptoms of depression are usually predominantly physical.

In the medical journal *CNS Spectrums*, doctors from the University of Medicine and Dentistry of New Jersey Robert Wood Johnson Medical School, Piscataway, NJ observe:

"Worldwide, patients with common mental disorders, such as depression and anxiety, have a tendency to present first to primary care exhibiting idiopathic [medically unexplained] physical symptoms. Typically, these symptoms consist of pain and other physical complaints that remain medically unexplained."

Thus, patients with depression who consult with a doctor complain of medically unexplained physical symptoms instead of psychological and emotional symptoms. For example, such patients say, "I have headaches" or "I'm tired all the time," rather than volunteering psychological symptoms such as, "Doctor, my mood is low and I'm depressed," or "I've lost interest in doing things," or "I'm nervous and anxious."

Depression and anxiety most often become recognizable by the associated, medically unexplained physical symptoms that a patient describes.

As you learned in the previous chapter,

The most common medically unexplained symptom associated with depression is pain.

Pain may involve a variety of areas: the head (headache), neck, back, chest, abdomen, pelvis, extremities, and widespread body ache. Other symptoms associated with depression include fatigue, insomnia, and change in body weight (gain or loss).

Chronic pain and depression are tightly linked.

Over one-half of depressed patients suffer from pain, and more than one in four patients who suffer from chronic pain report depression. *The Diagnostic and Statistical Manual of Mental Disorders* (DSM-IV) is the standard reference used by mental health professionals and doctors to classify and diagnose mental disorders. Written by the American Psychiatric Association (1994), it is based upon symptom description and categorization. Although DSM-V is anticipated in 2012, the criteria for diagnosis of depression in DSM-IV were revised in 2000 (DSM-IV-TR) to include bodily (somatic) symptoms as a symptom of depression. This reflects an increasing awareness of the association between physical symptoms and depression. These new criteria refer to "excessive worry over physical health and complaints of pain" (e.g., headaches or joint, abdominal, or other pains) among the associated features of major depressive disorder.

The Depression—Functional Somatic Syndromes Link

Chapter 5 introduced the concept of labeling collections of medically unexplained symptoms as symptom syndromes, called *functional somatic syndromes*. One example is fibromyalgia, a diagnostic label describing widespread bodily pain often accompanied by fatigue and sleep disturbance. Another is irritable bowel syndrome, which is the diagnosis made when abdominal pain is associated with disturbances of bowel function (diarrhea, constipation, or both). A recent medical review examining 244 studies confirms that there is a moderately strong association of depression and anxiety with functional somatic syndromes, including irritable bowel syndrome, functional dyspepsia, fibromyalgia, and chronic fatigue syndrome. Another medical journal article written by Drs. A. Tylee and P. Gandhi reinforces the syndrome—depression link:

"A holistic approach to recognition [of depression] is clearly necessary, and primary care physicians need to have a high index of suspicion for depression when faced with medically unexplained somatic symptoms, including general aches and pains and lack of energy."

Note that many of the physical symptoms of fibromyalgia are considered symptoms of depression. The core symptoms of functional somatic syndromes are chronic pain and discomfort associated with loss of vitality (fatigue, low energy, and sleep disturbance). These medically unexplained symptoms are also the most common symptoms of depression. Not only do the symptoms of functional somatic syndromes overlap with one another, they overlap and are associated with depression.

Medically Unexplained Symptoms "Predict" Diagnosis of Depression and Anxiety

Depression, anxiety, and somatoform disorders are the three most commonly associated psychiatric diagnoses in patients with medically unexplained symptoms (see Chapter 5). Indiana University's Dr. Kurt Kroenke and Judith

G. Rosmalen, PhD of the Department of Psychiatry, University Medical Center Groningen, University of Groningen, the Netherlands, collaborated to write a report about symptoms, syndromes, and psychiatric diagnoses in patients with medically unexplained symptoms. It was referenced in Chapter 4. They report that a depressive disorder can be diagnosed fifty to sixty percent of the time and an anxiety disorder forty to fifty percent of the time, regardless of symptom. Their findings reinforce three highly probable linkages between physical and emotional symptoms and syndromes.

1. If patients have symptoms that remain medically unexplained after evaluation, up to two-thirds have a depressive disorder, and up to one-half have an anxiety disorder.

    The specific type of symptom is not particularly important in terms of predicting depression or anxiety, but the number of symptoms is.

2. The greater the number of symptoms present, the greater the likelihood that depression and anxiety are associated.

    Among patients with zero to one symptom, four percent have associated depression or anxiety. For people having two to three symptoms, it is eighteen percent; for four to five, it is thirty-one percent; and for six to eight, it is fifty-two percent. If nine or more symptoms are present, seventy-eight percent of patients have associated anxiety or depression.

3. Medically unexplained physical symptoms are increasingly prevalent when patients experience severe psychological distress.

    Multiple unexplained physical symptoms are more likely in association with major depression than with minor depression or *dysthymia*. Dysthymia (or dysthymic disorder) is considered a less severe but longer-lasting depression. The presence of medically unexplained symptoms is lowest in those with no depression. The two symptoms most closely associated with depression are fatigue and insomnia, both of which are core symptoms of functional somatic syndromes. There is also a strong relationship between pain symptoms and depression.

Screening for Depression and Anxiety

In the *Journal of General Internal Medicine* in 1997, doctors report that depression can be identified by asking two simple questions. Asking them is particularly important when there are multiple, associated, medically unexplained symptoms. We think it is important for you to know these questions. You will find them in Dr. Kroenke's method for depression and anxiety screening, located in **PART 4** in the section on Learn How Doctors Think and Work with Them.

Are You a "Difficult Patient?"

Finally—and this will be difficult for most readers—as Dr. Kroenke and colleagues noted in Chapter 1 regarding the doctor/patient relationship, difficulty in the patient-physician encounter from the perspective of the doctor is a surprisingly good predictor of coexisting medically unexplained symptoms, depression, and/or anxiety. Primary care doctors consider approximately one out of every six outpatient visits to be difficult. Those patients they rate as difficult are two to three times more likely to have a depressive or anxiety disorder.

In sum, difficult doctor/patient encounters correlate strongly with both medically unexplained symptoms and the presence of multiple symptoms.

Now look closely at the stress association with disease and symptoms.

STRESS AND DISEASE/SYMPTOMS

You will learn much more about the epidemic of stress as you progress through the book. You will see stress differently.

For now, you know from your life experience how often you feel stressed out. You're not alone, because science confirms that most people feel this way most of the time.

Just as is the case with depression, science has also confirmed a powerful association of stress with serious disease. What we stated earlier bears repeating. Every element of metabolic syndrome, which include excess weight/obesity, high blood pressure, cholesterol abnormalities, elevated blood sugar and diabetes, and fatty liver can be promoted and/or aggravated by stress. Stress increases the risk of heart disease in healthy persons and increases the risk of dying in those who have had heart attacks. Stress is also associated with osteoporosis. Frankly, with the knowledge caregivers have regarding the link between stress and disease, we should be issuing the following warning:

When your body's stress response is constantly triggered, you may be vulnerable to serious health problems.

Stress is also linked to medically unexplained symptoms and functional somatic syndromes. The symptoms of stress ape other symptoms. Stress may be behind your headache, stomachache, lack of energy, and lower productivity. Its symptoms affect your thought processes, feelings, behaviors, and all of your body parts. You may not recognize the source of the problem, but you need to identify stress related issues in your life and take steps to deal with them.

Thoughts? Behaviors? Feelings? Are depression and stress linked? Can chronic stress cause depression? Is depression stressful?

While the cause of depression remains a complex subject, stress no doubt plays a part.

MEDICAL MELTDOWN REVISITED

Take another look at the medical meltdown. When a doctor considers your symptoms to be medically unexplainable, or labels collections of them as *functional somatic syndromes*, you must question whether depression and/or stress are their *cause*. You must look at the associations and linkages, but it is difficult to see and understand them.

Are you frustrated and/or dissatisfied? Are your doctors frustrated too? Is everyone's vision blurry?

Recall our discussion in Chapter 5 about how difficult it is for doctors to evaluate symptoms. Here's an example of the product of that dilemma. In his book, *Comfortably Numb*, Charles Barber explores medicalization and the medication of unhappiness. Seventy percent of the antidepressants sold throughout the world are sold in the United States. In 2006, 227 million antidepressant drug prescriptions were dispensed in the United States, more than any other class of medication. In that same year, the United States accounted for sixty-six percent of the global antidepressant market.

Remember, recent research confirms that:

Ten percent of the population is taking an antidepressant.

Are we more depressed here than people in the rest of the world? Are we trying harder to relieve medically unexplained symptoms that may be associated with depression? Are we under more stress? Or are we *medicalizing* life here more? If talk therapy for depression can be as effective—if not more effective—than drug use alone, do lower insurance coverage and higher out-of-pocket expenses for psychotherapy deter patients from seeing therapists and encourage taking an antidepressant pill?

Questions continue, as does the double hurt.

SPLITTING DOESN'T WORK

One of the main reasons we wrote this book is that:

Nothing in medicine is more confusing and frustrating for patients and doctors than the association of medically unexplained physical symptoms with depression and stress.

Most patients hurting from depression come to the doctor with medically unexplained physical symptoms. Assuming that the doctor recognizes the depression, neither the doctor nor the patient is likely to acknowledge and accept that the symptoms presented involve both the physical and the psychological. Patients feel invalidated and dismissed. They will say something like,

"You think this is all in my head, don't you?"

Doctors don't want to address the matter because even if they do understand it—and most don't—they do not have the time to explain or overcome the patient's foreseeable resistance. They might think, "The patient's not going to understand that the headaches are a somatic (bodily) expression of depression and/or stress. Anyway, I don't have time to explain it."

There is enough confusion, frustration, and misunderstanding surrounding these associations. If acknowledging the relationship of disease, symptoms, and syndromes with depression and stress weren't difficult enough, the degree of difficulty becomes even greater when trying to decipher cause and effect. For example,

The prevailing medical concept is that the most common "cause" of medically unexplained symptoms is undiagnosed depression, anxiety, and/or stress.

Do you remember when we asked you a question in the book's introduction?

"Is your view of your health and what's going on in the world of medicine blurry?"

Again, we reassure you that your vision is about to change.

SEE CLEARLY

Asking and answering all three questions that open this chapter will help you recognize that you hold the keys to self-discovery. We want you to see clearly that you do. We propose that the strong *association* of psychological/emotional symptoms and physical symptoms with depression and stress provides an opportunity for a new understanding and clearer vision as you proceed. In the **Illustrations** section at the beginning of the book, Figure 6.1 depicts three potential explanations or *causes* of the association. See these *causes* in Figure 6.1.

First, psychological/emotional symptoms reflecting a central (mind/brain) mechanism could be the cause of the physical symptoms.

"Doctor, are you saying that depression and stress are actually causing the pain?"

Second, psychological/emotional symptoms could be caused by the physical symptoms.

"Doctor, I'm depressed and stressed because of the pain!"

In either case, both patients and doctors are in a conceptual conundrum.

Is it mind/brain causing body hurt? Or does body hurt cause depression and stress?

Third, a potential explanation or cause can be understood by asking the correct question.

"What is behind the double hurt of mind/brain and body?"

The truth is, it's not an either/or matter. The *association* of depression and stress with disease, illness, medically unexplained symptoms, and symptom syndromes (functional somatic syndromes) is related to a *common cause*, which you will come to understand as you learn to ask new questions and begin the process of self-discovery. Now go back to the **Illustrations** section and look at Figure 6.2, which shows this very important concept that you will revisit in Chapter 13.

Here's an important clue regarding the identification of a common cause. In a medical review of the association of chronic pain and depression, Dr. Kroenke and colleagues write:

"Depression and pain share biological pathways and neurotransmitters, which has implications for the treatment of both concurrently. A model that incorporates assessment and treatment of depression and pain simultaneously is necessary for improved outcomes."

There is a common cause behind the associations and double hurt. While the cause includes stress and depression, it's much more complex, and understanding it demands a new way of looking at our problems. We promise that you won't finish our book without understanding it and seeing clearly.

MEDICATION AND TREATMENT

Once your vision is no longer blurry, you will be better able to partner with your doctor and other health care professionals in deciding that you might benefit by specific medications and treatments for your symptoms and/ or syndromes. You will learn more about your options in **PART 4:** Learn How Doctors Think and How to Work with Them.

LINK

For now, turn the pages, read, and reflect upon what most of us sense but don't talk about much. It's really a triple hurt.

CHAPTER 7

But It's Really a Triple Hurt for Most of Us

QUESTION

Why am I symptomatic?

QUOTE

"For this is the great error of our day in the treatment of the human being, that physicians separate the soul from the body."

The Dialogues of Plato, Vol. 1

PLATO

ABOUT THE QUOTE

Our collective professional experience has proved to us that the mind/brain, body, and external community are all inextricably linked.

In the quotation above, Plato articulates the ancient understanding that there is more to a person than material, physical being. For over two thousand years, long before the availability of scientific medicine, healers recognized that the health of a human being emerged from the harmonious, balanced relationships of a person's mind, body, and soul with his/her external environment. Symptoms, illness, and disease reflected disruptions of these relationships. Ancient healers did not have the wide range of prescription medications we have today. Instead, they relied upon helping people find their own ways to restore relationships. People understood this. But somewhere along the way, we lost this understanding. What we have not lost is the recognition that life is difficult and we are sick with symptoms.

CASE PRESENTATION: THE MINISTER/AUTHOR

The setting was a middle-school religion class in a suburban church I served. The topic was personal values. For openers, I asked the class to describe the standards and yardsticks they used to measure self-worth. Individually, but with some overlap, members of the class came up with the following list:

→ I am who I hang with;
→ I am what I belong to;
→ I am what I know;
→ I am what I do;
→ I am how I look;
→ I am what I have; and
→ I am how I act and behave.

Barely into their teens, they had already begun to define themselves by cultural norms. I noted that all their standards came from outside themselves, not from within. Specifically, they described peer status, group and team associations, grades, achievement, performance, fashion logos, dress size, others' expectations, and their ability to meet those expectations as the measuring rods for personal worth and success.

None of them identified anything close to a spiritual, intrinsic, or indwelling measurement of worth.

Throughout the discussion, they seemed dismayed and uncomfortable with the secular and extrinsic nature of their self-measurements. They talked about the pressure they felt to perform, keep up, and maintain appearances. They talked about feeling stressed. Among them was the hint of yearning. Something was missing. I felt they could sense it behind and underneath their symptomatic distress. I had my work cut out for me.

LOST...

In the introduction to *Care of the Soul: A Guide for Cultivating Depth and Sacredness in Everyday Life,* Thomas Moore writes:

The great malady...implicated in all our troubles and affecting us individually and socially is loss of soul...which appears symptomatically in obsession, addictions, violence, and loss of meaning...characterized by emptiness, meaninglessness, disillusionment, yearning, hunger for the spiritual, the sacred in our lives...

In a medical article, "Functional Illness in Primary Care: Dysfunction versus Disease," the authors write:

"Homo sapiens is body, mind, <u>and spirit</u>."

People have lost recognition of what the ancients knew. This is true whether people refer to their *inner lives* or use the language of *soul*. Internally disconnected and lacking meaningful relationships, they become symptomatic. You do, too.

...AND FOUND

The first chapter of Moore's book is entitled:

"Honoring Symptoms as a Voice of the Soul."

When symptomatic, you suffer the double hurt of mind/brain and body. It's really a triple hurt because the pain also involves your inner life, what many, like Moore, call "loss of soul." The double hurt and/or triple hurt epidemic demands your attention.

However, you look in the wrong direction when you focus solely upon the symptoms.

Instead, symptoms provide you with the opportunity to apply new science-based understanding that confirms the wisdom of ancient healing traditions. What has been lost can be found again. With rediscovery, you can learn how to nurture yourself by reintegrating mind/brain/body/soul relationships to find emergent health.

INTEGRATIVE MEDICINE

Many academic medical centers now advocate the integration of the best of scientific medicine with alternative and complementary therapies that address the whole person, including mind/brain, body, spirit, and community. Examples include the University of Arizona's Arizona Center for Integrative Medicine, founded and co-directed by Andrew Weil, M.D., and Duke University's Duke Integrative Medicine. Consider exploring the resources each provides.

LINK

Conclude your study of **PART 1: The Epidemic of Symptoms** by reading and reflecting upon the next chapter, where you will begin to find that YOU, rather than your diagnosis or diagnoses, determine your health.

CHAPTER 8

The Diagnosis Doesn't Determine YOUR Health; YOU Do

QUESTIONS

I've been diagnosed with ___, but I feel something's been left unsaid in the diagnosis.

What's missing?
What am I missing?
What isn't being said?

QUOTE

"You've always had the power to go back to Kansas."

Glinda the Good Witch to Dorothy
The Wonderful Wizard of Oz
L. FRANK BAUM

ABOUT THE QUOTE

Use the new understanding we have provided to remind yourself of the power within you to imagine your well-being and health. It is your creative responsibility.

To limit yourself by diagnostic labels and see yourself only as a consumer of health care products and treatment is to miss the vital link in your own self-care.

Begin your exploration here.

CASE PRESENTATION: DOCTOR/AUTHOR

A.T. is a fifty-two-year-old married executive secretary who consulted me for lower abdominal pain, intermittent diarrhea and constipation, abdominal bloating, and nausea. She admitted that the symptoms had troubled her since her teenage years and that they came and went. She decided to come in because the symptoms had been especially bad over the past six months. She had gained about thirty pounds over the past year, even though she reported that she wasn't eating very much. She slept poorly and was tired all of the time. She hurt all over and felt unwell. Several doctors had made diagnoses of irritable bowel syndrome, fibromyalgia syndrome, chronic tension headache, temporomandibular joint disorder, and depression. Despite these diagnoses and treatments, she was still sick.

I directed four questions to her.

1. "What is going on in your life now and how are you feeling about it?"
2. "What do you think is wrong with you?"
3. "What are you worried might be wrong with you?"
4. "What is your self-care plan?"

She responded that there was a lot of stress. She thought that her symptoms might be related to "it." She wasn't sure why she had these symptoms, and she was worried that she might have cancer or another serious disease. Finally, she admitted that she had no self-care plan.

Her physical examination was normal except that her blood pressure was slightly high. Blood tests showed a mild elevation of fasting blood sugar and that her cholesterol profile was abnormal. A colonoscopy showed no abnormalities to explain her symptoms.

I reassured her that her symptoms were real, but not indicative of a serious or life-threatening disease. I briefly explained the labeling process of medicalization and generating symptoms through disconnections and imbalance and gave her educational materials to read and study. I also recommended several books. I indicated that she had early metabolic syndrome, an increased risk of diabetes and heart disease, and advised her to develop a self-care plan.

She did not return for over a year. When she did, she came primarily to express her appreciation and explain that she had linked her symptoms and health problems to a difficult relationship in her life. She was no longer sick. She had a self-care plan that included exercise, healthy diet, and yoga. She had lost the weight that she had gained and confirmed that her blood pressure, blood sugar, and cholesterol values improved once she divorced her husband. She had also rediscovered her faith in God.

THE MISSING LINK

When you are symptomatic and a doctor diagnoses your symptoms as *syndromatic*, the syndrome by itself neither defines the root cause of your symptoms nor predetermines a probable outcome. It is merely the name given to a collection of symptoms that have no medically explainable cause. This is a great frustration to physicians who have been trained to think about cause and effect in a linear manner. Diffuse, non-linear, unexplainable symptoms don't fit that style of thinking.

When tests fail to provide a medical explanation for your aches and pains, the only recourse is to label them.

You may feel some relief by having a medical name given to what ails you, but in truth, all you've received is a label that doesn't bring much relief. Now you are stuck with the label medically because doctors don't like to treat what they cannot test for or explain. The tag you've been given will not easily come off. Sooner or later, you will become frustrated, too. Symptoms persist. You are not getting better. You may feel worse.

Read again the questions that introduce this chapter.

You question what's missing and isn't being said. You are right in asking these questions. They are the right questions to ask. However, the answer to, "What's missing and isn't being said?" is a paradox. What is missing when you are symptomatic is you. We mean by this the whole you, the one who is greater than the sum of your body parts and bodily functions.

HOW CAN THIS BE TRUE?

You might be wondering, "How can this be true?" You're the patient. You're the one being examined and diagnosed. How can you be "what's missing" in your own treatment and care? The reasons are complex and multi-layered. Unraveling them requires patience, perseverance, and willingness to suspend belief in notions about health care you have taken for granted.

Then you can begin to unlearn what you have assumed to be givens and rediscover the focus of ancient healing and wisdom traditions.

It is the whole self.

None of this is easy. What you believe and take for granted regarding your personal health and well-being may be ingrained in family values and passed down wisdom, religious dogma, your own experience, and community lore. What you actually practice may vary from what you believe. You smoke, knowing it's not good for you, or you don't get enough exercise. You find your habits compromising your better sense of self while New Year's resolutions fade into January gray. You feel stuck. You wonder why.

LIFE IS HARD, TOO FAST, COMPLICATED, AND VERY STRESSFUL. YOU WEREN'T DESIGNED TO LIVE THIS WAY, SO YOU'RE SYMPTOMATIC

From experience, you agree. Getting by is its own necessity. You're tired at the end of the day. The hurry and rush does not leave much time for reflection. Work-numb, maybe you find it easier to flip through *Real Simple* or flip on cable TV. Perhaps you surf the web or answer e-mail until you go to bed. Besides, it's hard trying to wade through all the stuff about what and why you believe what you do regarding your own health and well-being.

Life learning is a messy process.

Self-perception is often shaded and skewed by things known and unknown. Like the rest of us, you perceive that there are many facets to personhood. Some you like. They are lustrous. Others are shadowy and unconscious. You don't talk about them much. Masked and repressed, they don't see the light of day. Thoughts, feelings, and pent-up emotion go unexpressed. Instead, your symptoms do the talking.

FIX ME, I'M BROKEN

Ironically, the existence and treatment of symptoms provide a link between you and all who are symptomatic and receiving care. The irony is that the linkage is actually a shared misconception. The misconception is that personal health care is something to be received, employed, and consumed. That is, the doctor's or other caregiver's office is a repair shop.

"Fix me, I'm broken," the patient as consumerist thinks.

From our professional interaction with peers, this perception appears to hold true, regardless of the type of care being rendered, be it medical, psychological, spiritual, or some alternative.

FIXED BY WHOM?

Dr. Paul W. Pruyser was a clinical psychologist and coauthor of Dr. Menninger's book, *The Vital Balance*. In his book, *Minister as Diagnostician: Personal Problems in Pastoral Perspective*, he asks, "For all human misfortunes, difficulties, mishaps, or symptoms presented to the various helping professions, how does one find out what the problem is?"

Dr. Pruyser writes that each specialist pushes for his own viewpoint of the problem. Who's the fixer?

Are you beginning to identify who the "fixers" are in your life and who really holds the key to discovering what's behind your symptoms?

FINDING THE INTERNAL TRUTH

One premise underlying the "fix me, I'm broken" care model is that personal health only comes from outside one's self and not from within. The opposite is true. Within you lies the physical, mental, and spiritual power to fuel your own journey toward healthful well-being.

The body is capable of effecting its own healing. The mind/brain is able to change and retune itself (in medical language, this is called *neuroplasticity*). The soul or inner life is able to uplift, enlighten, and reintegrate a whole sense of self.

All of this is possible from within.

THE BIG PROBLEM

However, there's a problem. Most people don't know or believe this to be true. They have never learned or have misplaced along the way the idea that a person has the intrinsic ability to generate his or her own health. How can this be? Again, the reasons are multi-layered. Let's try to pick away at the lack of understanding from the outer to the inner layers.

PROBLEMS WITH MEDICINE AND HEALTH CARE

To begin, we will be blunt.

In our current health care model, many medical professionals lack the training, time, and inclination to deal with you holistically. Yet it is the whole you that needs to be engaged.

Testing body functions doesn't do that. Examining different body parts specialist by specialist doesn't do that. Time constraints leave much unsaid. Functional analysis trumps discernment of the whole. While hopeful trends are emerging among some health care professionals who emphasize the patient's personal ownership of health care management, the prevalent theme remains consumerist.

"Fix me, Doc; I'm broken."

And so, you are still hurting.

PROBLEMS WITH COMPLEMENTARY AND ALTERNATIVE MEDICINE

In response or reaction to the linear thinking limitations of the medical care model, alternative forms of therapy and treatment have become popular. They run the homeopathic, chiropractic, meditative, physical, and spiritual development gamut. Many provide helpful discipline in dealing with a person's self-care. Yet often, they too reinforce the mindset of consumer in the product user or treatment receiver. "If I use this product, I'll lose weight, sleep better, feel peppier, cease to ache," the product user surmises. "If I follow this treatment discipline or allow my body to be manipulated just so, my back won't hurt and I won't feel so stressed," the follower of the discipline seeks to believe. In part, this may be true. Again, however, there is a tendency to piecemeal one's sense of well-being, get parts relating—mental, physical, or spiritual—without connecting and integrating the whole person.

As in medicine, these disciplines, treatments, and products do not provide cross-integration.

Seeing three medical specialists for three diverse sets of symptoms usually guarantees that none of them will evaluate and integrate all the symptoms. Your Pilates instructor will not have direct contact with your chiropractor, nor will a health foods retailer discuss homeopathic alternatives with your doctor's nurse. St. John's wort and ginkgo biloba may sit in your medicine cabinet next to the aspirin and prescription medicine. Unless you've raised the question with a pharmacist or physician, you don't know how they interact.

PROBLEMS WITH MENTAL HEALTH CARE

If you are seeing a psychiatrist, psychologist, or psychoanalyst, he or she cannot talk to other caregivers in your life unless you consent. You may not want anyone to know you're seeing one. And if you're depressed, what about all of those distressing bodily symptoms? Where do they fit in? In medicine, alternative medicine, and mental health care, there is a singular constant.

The constant is YOU.

If you are fragmented, symptomatic, and seemingly stuck with a fix me mindset, you don't have the big picture regarding your well-being and care. No one else appears to have one, either, because they are not treating the whole you. Where else can you look for the answers?

PROBLEMS WITH SPIRITUAL CARE

Searching for a larger frame of reference, perhaps you explore a new spiritual discipline or worship in a temple, mosque, or church. There you seek respite and insight. Conceptually, religion ("to bring together, bind up") is all about the big picture: creation, life forces, the universe, life journeys, and where human beings fit into the scene. When true to its big-picture roots, religion may inspire by helping you think holistically. At its best, it may comfort you when you are hurt and discomfort you when you have become too comfortable with your own material status, ambition, perfectionism, or malaise.

These days, however, you need to listen carefully to what any spiritual belief system proffers as its core message.

If the message sounds small (as in small-minded, small godly, clannish, and exclusive), it likely is. Does the message giver raise the right questions or claim to have all the right answers? *Answer* faiths abound. They play on both their collective need and the individuals' personal yearning for black and white clarity in a messy learning, difficult world. Rarely will they have much investment in helping you seek out and raise the *right* questions for your personal journey. Instead, they will be loaded with the *right* answers about what to believe and how to behave to be acceptable, accepted, and/or saved. In this vein, such belief systems are simply a spiritual variation of the "fix me; I'm broken" mindset. They tie your need to be fixed with their need to be exclusive fixers.

Lost in all this is the reality that life is difficult, not simplistic.

Life learning is a messy process, not a linear, literal reading of religious ABCs. When the message is reduced to small-minded pat answers, other things are lost as well. One is an integrated, holistic world view. Another is the whole you.

This is spiritual repair shop religion.

Its working premise is to serve as religious *fixer*. Like medicine when practiced *on the clock*, repair shop religion has a hard time thinking inventively. Small minds that adhere to their own brand of linear thinking shrink the big picture. They have no room for the unexplainable, the hard questions, and accompanying doubts. When you are symptomatic, they may have all the pre-packaged *answers*, but there is really no wandering, wondering breathing space for you.

EXPLORE AND RETURN TO POWER

If you are like most people and have experienced the fragmented, repair shop care we have been describing, you may be asking yourself,

So now what do I do?

First,

Understand that we are trying, from our professional vantage points, to inform you of the limitations and disadvantages of core understandings of modern health care delivery, such as medicalization. They are serious.

As we will discuss further, the linear thinking of health care providers does not connect all the dots when you are symptomatic. Because your care is fragmented, you may remain fragmented. Often your care is rudderless as well, with no single professional caregiver at the helm.

Second,

Reread the quote that begins this chapter.

As Glinda advised Dorothy, she always had the power to go home again; she just had to learn it for herself. Through self-exploration, you have the power to find what ancient healing traditions have always known. Your health is not about fragmentation. Instead, it's about integration of mind, body, and soul; it's all about connections, balance, and relationships.

Third,

Ask questions of yourself and your caregivers: "What's behind the symptoms?"

As Elliott Dacher, M.D., writes in his book, *Intentional Healing*:

"The first stage of healing always begins with breakdown. The first stage of healing is characterized by a focus on, and attention to, the external manifestations of distress (symptoms)."

Fourth,

Read on.

Your care does not have to be managed like this. You are not fated to be symptomatic and forever sick. You can take charge of your own health and well-being. It's now time for you to begin to find answers to the question, "What is behind the symptoms?"

LINK

You're ready to learn how to begin the process of imagining your own wellness. Turn the page and discover in **PART 2** how the balanced self is intended to work.

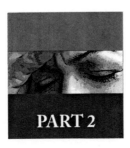

The Balanced Self

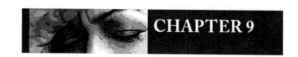

CHAPTER 9

The Complexity of YOUR Life and YOUR Health

QUESTION

What is good health?

QUOTES

"Patients are angry by implicitly being labeled as not having a 'real' disease and not getting a satisfactory explanation for why they suffer from their symptoms."

Gastroenterology (June, 2008)
EMERAN A. MAYER, M.D.
Gastroenterologist and Executive Director, UCLA Center for Neurobiology of Stress

"I came to fully understand that the mind and the body were one—not separated, not disconnected. What affected one also affected the other."

Symptoms of Unknown Origin: A Medical Odyssey
CLIFTON K. MEADOR, M.D.
Clinical Professor of Medicine, Vanderbilt School of Medicine

"The whole is more than the sum of its parts."

Aristotle's Metaphysics
ARISTOTLE

ABOUT THE QUOTES

Edward Sarafino's textbook, *Health Psychology: Biopsychosocial Interactions*, opens with two questions:

"You know what health is, don't you?"

"How would you define it?"

In the pages that follow, you will learn to answer them for yourself. For now, **PART 2** of this book is about you and the systems relationships, both internal and environmental, from which balance and health—both good and bad—emerge.

CASE PRESENTATION

N.J. is a sixty-three-year-old friend of ours who considers himself to be in good health. While he doesn't have any symptoms of concern, he admits to having occasional headaches, indigestion, and insomnia. He usually sees his doctor only for preventative care. He recognizes that his health depends upon the relationship between the internal environment of his body and the external environment of the world. He knows that his health related behavior is very important. Therefore, he has imagined himself well and created a good self-care plan, including eating a Mediterranean diet, maintaining a healthy weight, exercising regularly, and reducing stress through meditation, positive attitude, and trying to avoid high demand – low control stressors.

THE LIMITATIONS OF MODERN MEDICINE

At this point in your reading, you've already learned a hard, dismaying lesson. Modern medicine cannot account for the epidemic of symptoms and syndromes that are medically unexplained. Nor can it treat linearly the association between depression and/or stress and patients' symptoms. The consequences for both patients and caregivers are confusion, dissatisfaction, and frustration. Fragmentation of care is the rule, not the exception.

Everyone hurts.

You still suffer and that hurts.

THE BIOMEDICAL MODEL OF HEALTH DOESN'T WORK

Regardless of its limitations, the model of care that has been applied by health care professionals for the past 300 years remains prevalent, even though it doesn't work very well. As the name implies, the biomedical model continues to maintain that all illness can be medically explained biologically. This includes genetic predispositions and environmental factors. It assumes that any psychological causative influence is a secondary factor. The biomedical model holds onto the premise that the mind and body function as separate entities. It insists upon separation of the mind and body, even though it:

→ cannot explain illness without disease;
→ cannot explain depression and symptom association;
→ emphasizes treatment of illness and disease over the promotion of health; and
→ views health as the absence of disease.

This model limits itself to a one-dimensional, evaluative approach to which it is predisposed. What it wants to test and account for is the presence or absence of disease. While it does consider the fact that environmental factors may influence or alter the nature and severity of disease, it has little clinical diagnostic appreciation for subjective perceptions (illness) or psychological influences. Any *psychological overlay* (note that this is a pejorative medical term) is at best a secondary factor, and illness is accounted for by the clinical diagnosis of disease.

Notice what doesn't fit within the model at all: it is illness without disease, the prime example of which is the presence of medically unexplained symptoms and/or syndromes.

Let's quickly review why this is the case.

Two problematic assumptions prop up the biomedical model. The first, known as *reductionism*, proposes that diagnosis of symptomatic conditions is a matter of linear cause and effect. (A), the symptoms, are caused by (B), the diagnosis, as confirmed by medical tests. You already know the weaknesses of this narrow approach.

The second questionable premise is the tendency of physicians to evaluate and *split* your symptoms into two categories—disease or illness. Disease, you'll remember, is definable and causatively verifiable. It is organic. On the other hand, illness is subjective. It is your perception of poor health, which is evidenced by your symptom reports and health-related behavior. It has no explainable cause. It is functional, as your doctor puts it—psychosomatic as your doctor may think it—because it cannot be confirmed by medical testing.

Not just patients are angry over the splitting and labeling. The categorizing angers and frustrates caring professionals as well.

From a personal perspective, both of us have used our distress, frustration, and empathy as motivation for writing this book. In the case of gastroenterology, Dr. Emeran Mayer, gastroenterologist and the author of the first quote of this chapter writes:

"The traditional model of separating 'functional' from 'organic' disorders of the gastrointestinal (GI) tract has not been helpful for patients, their physicians, or investigators."

While this evaluative approach fits neatly into the cubicles and boundaries of modern medicine, it really doesn't work well in advancing the cause of discovering why you feel the way you do. As you know from personal experience and by reading this far, disease and illness don't separate themselves neatly into two distinct categories. You can have disease with illness. You can have disease without illness. Mysteriously, you can suffer illness without disease. The inexplicability of that is the Achilles heel of modern medical care. Because your medically unexplained symptoms (MUS) cannot be reduced or neatly boxed, the biomedical model doesn't work.

INTERRELATING MODELS THAT DO WORK

Fortunately, there are interconnected systems models that do provide a useful framework of understanding. They are the biopsychosocial model, the holistic model of ancient healers, and the new model of homeostasis and allostasis, which confirms ancient wisdom.

The Biopsychosocial Model

In 1977, Dr. George Engel of the University of Rochester proposed a new medical model. His article, "The Need for a New Medical Model: The Challenge for Biomedicine," published in *Science*, outlines what Dr. Engel describes as a *biopsychosocial model* of disease and illness. Under this model, multiple factors influence and affect your health:

→ **Bio**logical (anatomic and physiologic);
→ **Psycho**logical (thoughts, memories, beliefs, attitudes, emotions, and feelings);
→ **Social** (interpersonal relationships).

One of us (WBS) had not understood the significance of this model until he studied the teachings of gastroenterologist Douglas A. Drossman, M.D., Professor of Medicine and Psychiatry at the University of North Carolina School of Medicine, who was one of Dr. Engel's students and is a world-renowned expert in irritable bowel syndrome and functional

GI syndromes. What became evident is that the biopsychosocial model rightly comprehends that early life influences (genetics and environment, both physical and social) affect you psychosocially and biologically. They influence your behaviors, the way you function, and your health. They can be key contributors to your being symptomatic. While the biopsychosocial model is complex, what's important for you to understand is that YOU are complex.

Your symptoms, especially medically unexplained symptoms, are expressions of altered mind/brain and bodily function that may be the consequence of multiple factors.

For example, depending upon your inherited genetic predispositions (temperament and vulnerability factors), the experience of high levels of stress, emotional distress (anxiety or depression), lack of social support, and physical/biochemical changes in your body interact down to the cellular level to affect your health and produce illness and disease. Various personal, interpersonal, and social factors affect your health for good and ill. Given the interactive interplay, mind and body are not separate, as they are in the biomedical model. Both intimately relate to issues of disease and illness. Both influence the state of your health, along with the external and inner life or *soulful* influences at work around and within you.

As you learned in Chapter 4, WBS had a teacher at Vanderbilt University Hospitals who inspired him to care for the patient and look behind the symptom. Dr. Clifton Meador is the author of the second quote that introduces this chapter. In his book, *Symptoms of Unknown Origin: A Medical Odyssey*, he writes of his understanding around the time that Dr. Engel's biopsychosocial model was published:

I came to fully understand that the mind and the body were one—not separated, not disconnected. What affected one also affected the other. Sitting above all the molecules, tissues, organs, and mind of the human body was an integrated person. This person was connected to a family and perhaps to a spouse, and the family was connected to some social structure and society at large. All this social structure impinged on the person, and the person impinged on the social structure. There was a continuum all the way from society to the person to the organs and even down to the molecules. There were no separated pockets or islands. There certainly was no mind separated from a body.

Sounds reasonable, doesn't it? Haven't you found that a variety of factors is at work in your life, influencing the way you think and feel? Recognizing that various influences affect your health, the model fits the facts. Nevertheless, as a standalone theory, the biopsychosocial model suffers from several debilities, one of which we will address in Chapter 11. For now, we'll call the model's first debility an absence of awareness issue.

Many caregivers and most patients don't know what the biopsychosocial model is.

You will most likely never hear the term used during health care treatment. Exacerbating the model's public relations problem is that it attempts to take a big picture look at your health in what is otherwise a myopic, piecemeal, and fragmented care arena. Given the prevalence of the reductionist biomedical model, the biopsychosocial model lacks market share influence. In addition, even its proponents often fail to raise two critical pieces of inquiry when you are symptomatic.

First, they do not explore your question:

How are these multiple factors generating my symptoms?

Second, they do not emphasize your need to ask:

What's behind my symptoms and why am I symptomatic?

While both questions are critical to your self-understanding, they are not raised. Why? You already know the answer. The biopsychosocial model suffers from a problem you've encountered throughout your own care.

There's not enough time for in-depth patient/doctor discussion.

Even when doctors and other care professionals understand the model, they don't often employ it. It's too time consuming and impractical to get at all the multiple biological, psychological, and social factors that could be influencing your health. The quick fix is preferable to searching for, raising, and discussing all the possible right questions. It's easier for the doctor to prescribe a drug. It's easier for you, the patient, to take it. Just because it's easier doesn't mean you're healed. In fact, you're still hurting. While the biopsychosocial model provides helpful perspective in seeing the bigger picture regarding your health, it is not a cure-all. An additional key question remains unstated:

How are my symptoms and daily life issues connected?

On all of these matters, there is silence. You need help in asking and answering them. But the care giving disciplines are too disjointed; and most doctors stuck in a biomedical model of care won't be inclined to raise these questions or help you answer them. You need self-care assistance. You need a complementary model to assist you in finding health. It's available. We've already referred to it. And it's been around a long time. Here is where you will begin to see clearly.

The Holistic Model of the Ancient Healers

Among diverse societies, from ancient Greek to Chinese, Indian to Native American, caregivers and care receivers believed in holistic health. Key to their practices and beliefs was their reverence for the following concept: personal health depended upon both internal and external harmony. Internal stability involved mind/body/inner life integration. External harmony with the environment was also necessary. Health emerged when both were in balance. Symptoms and disease emerged when these relationships were disrupted and fractured.

Drawing upon their holistic perspective, the ancients raised and answered the questions that modern caregivers have failed to address. Seeing a whole person who interacts with all of his or her surroundings, they helped the person to look behind the symptoms to uncover what was generating them.

There, some people found internal fracture—mind/body/inner life not in sync. Others found themselves out of rhythm and harmony with their environments. Whatever they found, their healers did not try to fix or repair one part of the body in isolation from the whole. Instead, they sought to restore the whole, which was fractured internally and/or externally. Critical to healing was the appraisal of a person's life and health in a comprehensive and integrated way.

Remember Aristotle's quote at the beginning of the chapter?

"The whole is more than the sum of its parts."

That's what the ancients believed. We do, too. The whole of you is greater than the sum of your individual parts. As you will see in the next chapter, body parts are important. However, what constitutes life and the living of it is much more than the cells, molecules, tissue, and organs of which you are composed. It is the integration, interaction, and interrelationship of the parts that make you YOU, which make you tick, and when you are out of sync, make you symptomatic and sick. Science has confirmed the wisdom of the ancient healing traditions.

The Body's Natural Balancing System:
Homeostasis and Allostasis

In *The Wisdom of the Body*, first published in 1939, Dr. Walter B. Cannon recognizes that natural processes of your body are set up to maintain optimal physiological balance. This is known as *homeostasis*. Furthermore, he explains that to keep this balance, the mind/brain must receive information input that constantly reports the status and condition of all of the tissues of the body. For Dr. Cannon, homeostasis is a dynamic, ongoing process that involves multiple interrelated systems whose primary purpose is your survival and health.

In 1988, Peter Sterling and Joseph Eyer of the University of Pennsylvania named the homeostatic process *allostasis* in the *Handbook of Life Stress, Cognition, and Health*. Allostasis is the mind/brain and body's ability to achieve stability through and despite change. This dynamic process is critical for your survival.

Any threat or change triggers an allostatic stabilizing response. Like a rocking teeter-totter, the allostatic process is in constant motion, responding to change and threat. This occurs whether the changes and threats are real or not and whether you are consciously aware of them or not.

Threat and change are referred to collectively as *stressors*.

They are the totality of all that presents itself to you in the world around you, and on which you may place the blame if life becomes overwhelming. Less obvious is that you have stressors within the internal environment of your mind/brain and body.

We refer to physical stressors—the tangible and measurable stressors—as *the tiger in your path*:

→ Accident/trauma
→ Alcohol in excess
→ Circadian light-dark cycle/rhythms
→ Food
→ Infection/virus
→ Injury
→ Medication
→ Seasonal change
→ Poison
→ Surgery
→ Temperature extremes
→ Tobacco
→ Toxin
→ Travel

We refer to psychological stressors, the intangible and/or immeasurable, as *the tiger in your mind*:

→ Interpersonal and relational issues (home, work, community)
→ Loss (e.g., job, divorce, death)
→ Major life events

→ Post-traumatic responses
→ Medical disease
→ Menstruation
→ Menopause
→ Mid-life crisis
→ Anxiety
→ Depression

Think about the physical and psychological "tiger" stressors in your life.

What's going on within the internal environment of your mind/brain and body can be stressful!

But being *stressed* is much more than being exposed to stressors.

THE STRESS RESPONSE

While stressors such as major life events and trauma receive the emphasis, what is really important is your *stress response* to environmental factors. You will study the environmental factors, both internal and external, throughout the rest of the book.

So, from this point on, when we refer to stress, we really mean *the stress response*.

The stress response (allostasis) emerges as an adaptation to stressors regardless of their source. These can be psychologically traumatic experiences and/or physically traumatic experiences like an invasion of the body by infection/virus.

While the original stressor may be temporary and self-limited, the stress response may be ongoing. Its persistence may contribute to your symptoms.

Many people constantly feel stressed, but you might be one of those folks who don't feel anxious or stressed very often. You wonder how all of this could be related to your symptoms. The reality is that stress may be activated without any conscious awareness that you are feeling stressed.

We also call unconscious stress *the crouching tiger in your mind*.

The tiger is lurking, whether you are aware of it or not.

STRESS IS A PARADOX: BOTH GOOD AND BAD

Dr. Bruce S. McEwen at Rockefeller University in New York is considered one of the world's authorities on stress. In his book, *The End of Stress as*

We Know It, Dr. McEwen writes that there's a new way to think about and understand stress. Part of that understanding is as follows:

Stressor
→ Any threat or change to homeostasis, real or perceived
→ Perception is influenced by experiences, genetics, and behavior

Stress Response
→ Allostasis = *Good Stress*
→ Allostatic load = *Bad Stress*

As you continue reading, keep both good stress and bad stress in mind. Both influence your well-being, and as you will see in **PART 3,** bad stress is a pivotal component in poor health.

Given the layered complexity of your whole self and the necessary interconnection of the three models we have just discussed, you can begin to understand why a narrow, one-dimensional, linear approach to diagnosing your symptoms doesn't work effectively. This is particularly true when your doctors cannot confirm or explain their cause. A shift in perspective is in order.

To FIND HEALTH, YOU need to be the one to do it.

Doctors and other caring professionals are your resources.

THE NECESSARY SHIFT FROM LINEAR
TO NONLINEAR PERSPECTIVE

In a complex world, with its uncertainty, nuance, and shades of gray, it is understandable why you might yearn for things to be black or white. It would make life simpler, easier to evaluate and to understand. The same is true for medicine. Seeking to sail safely around the Symptoms Iceberg, doctors prefer linear diagnostic navigation. It is less time-consuming and more efficient to practice medicine if a straightforward rule of cause and effect applies. The symptoms (A) are caused by the diagnosis (B). The stimulus and response are proportionate. The severity of the symptoms reflects the degree of seriousness of their cause.

Think of the linear perspective of cause and effect as a supposedly clear direct line between disease/diagnosis and symptoms. Seeking clarity, it settles for being myopic. The resulting diagnosis is piecemeal. There is no big picture to provide perspective and assessment of the whole you. This approach is roughly analogous to trying to comprehend the whole of a large machine by disassembling it to study its parts. In the process, you miss the whole of what it is because the whole is greater than the sum of its parts. The same holds true when doctors use a linear approach to diagnose what's wrong with you.

Compounding the problem is the fact that the world is full of complex systems that do not lend themselves to linear causal explanation.

A human being is one such complex system. Never forget that you are layered.

These systems cannot be understood simply by analyzing their individual parts. While the parts are important, their integration and interrelationships are even more so. Within them cause and effect is neither straightforward nor proportionate. As you know from your own life, small systemic changes can have major effects. A different perspective is necessary to understand how they work.

In contrast, a circular, swirling design of mutually interactive relationships between disease/diagnosis and symptoms reflects life in holistic perspective. There is flowing interaction among the parts of the whole. That interaction is a key to understanding the whole system. You may remember the Wendy's ad with the catch phrase "Parts is parts." The commercial played upon what made up their competitor's chicken nuggets and fingers. While Wendy's was cleverly selling the quality of its fast food, the ad line contained an underlying, if unintended, truth applicable to more than just chicken.

Parts are just parts in any complex system. How they interact is what gives the system life.

It's the interaction that is the key.

LIFE AND THE SCIENCE OF COMPLEXITY

Reflect upon what it means to believe that,

"The whole is more than the sum of its parts."

While it is not our intent to immerse you (and likely lose you as a reader) in complexity science and complex systems theory (take a quick look at some of the references in the **Bibliography**), there are several reference points for you to keep in mind:

→ *Complexity science* is a non-linear holistic discipline that attempts to understand the nature of the interaction of complicated systems, including human life.

→ *Complex adaptive systems* are systems composed of many interacting parts that learn, evolve and adapt over time. They are complex and flexible. The loss of complexity and flexibility results in *decomplexification* and inflexibility. In the mind/brain and body, this loss can mean chronic pain, symptoms, disease, and even death.

→ *Relationship* is a key concept in complexity science. It refers to the interconnections between and among parts of a system that are as or more important than the component parts themselves. For example, you have billions of brain cells, called *neurons*. Individual neurons are incapable of thought. Fortunately, for thoughtful people like you, neurons are interrelated and interact with one another. (See concept of *emergence* below.)

→ *Non-linear behavior* refers to the fact that the magnitude of response is not necessarily proportional to the intensity of the stimulus. This is known as *the butterfly effect*, which is attributed to mathematician and meteorologist Edward Lorenz, a pioneer in chaos (complexity) theory. To emphasize this effect, one of his lectures to the Association for the Advancement of Science in 1972 bears the title, "Does the Flap of a Butterfly's Wings in Brazil Set off a Tornado in Texas?"

→ *Decentralization* means that there is self-organization without a leader. The advantage is that the system can be *smarter* in learning and adapting than its smartest part.

→ *Emergence* is the term used for the process of pattern formation in a complex system. The pattern is formed from basic component parts or behaviors. The parts do not simply coexist. They relate and interact. Following the previous example, the relationships and interactions of those billions of neurons result in a brain capable of thought. Because they interact, you can think; and your ability to think is much greater than the sum of all those billions of neurons.

→ **You are a *complex adaptive system*.** Actually, you are composed of various *complex adaptive systems* (for example, the mind/brain, within which are many subsystems). The systems are adaptive because they have the ability to learn from prior experience, acclimate to changing environments, make modifications, change, and evolve. What is true for each system within you is also true for the whole you. You can change and find health.

From this brief survey, you begin to see that contemporary scientific inquiry is exploring territory already familiar to you. You may not describe what you know in complexity science terms. Yet from gut feelings, inner life activity, spiritual yearnings, subconscious thoughts, philosophical questions, psychological insights, social interactions, or all of the above,

You already know that living your life is multi-layered and complex.

Whatever your desire for simplicity, less stress, and clear sailing, you are a complex, adaptive being living in an interactive, complex world. In his book, Dr Meador writes:

I want to make it as clear as I possibly can that this book is not a criticism of scientific reductionism. I am in awe of the method and its effectiveness. My point here is that scientific reduction is not the same process as clinical medicine. It is the sheer scientific power of the biomedical model that has blinded so many as to its clinical limitations and restrictions.

We agree. We intend that you not be blinded but see clearly. We will share more wisdom from Dr. Meador in **PART 4**.

THE NECESSARY VIEW OF HOLISM

From a holistic perspective, you now see the internal environment of your mind/brain-body as a complex adaptive system comprised of many complex adaptive systems living within and interacting with the complex adaptive systems of the external environment. The ancients were correct, because the whole is so much more than the sum of its parts.

Complexity science forms the scientific basis of holism.

While great scientific progress has been made through reductionist research, holism and complexity theory are the new views that are revolutionizing scientific research in multiple disciplines. This is the continuing lesson of **PART 2**. Chapter 10 will concentrate on your internal environment, Chapter 11 on the world around you, and Chapter 12 on your spiritual inner life. Here you will learn how you are mapped out for health.

LINK

Prepare yourself to compare and contrast the rest of **PART 2** with **PART 3**, in which we will describe how the very systems meant for health can produce symptoms, illness, hurt, and disease when they are out of balance.

CHAPTER 10

How YOU Emerge: Balance and YOUR Internal Environment

QUESTIONS

How do the mind/brain and body relate and communicate with one another? Why do I need to know, anyway?

QUOTES

"We are returning to original beliefs that the mind and body cannot be separated."

Timeless Healing: The Power and Biology of Belief
HERBERT BENSON, M.D.

"Research now shows that your brain is teeming with body maps—maps of your body's surface, its musculature, its intentions, its potential for action, even a map that automatically tracks and emulates the actions of other people around you."

The Body Has a Mind of Its Own
SANDRA BLAKESLEE and MATTHEW BLAKESLEE

"As a man thinks (within himself) so is he."

Proverbs 23: 7

ABOUT THE QUOTES

We introduced you to Dr. Herbert Benson in Chapter 6. Here he asserts that ancient healing traditions had it right: you cannot understand personal health, disease, illness, and healing without appreciating the connection between the mind/brain and the body. Dr. Benson's book emphasizes the relationship between faith and the mind and body's health. Sandra Blakeslee, science writer for *The New York Times*, and her son, Matthew Blakeslee, bring a different perspective by looking at the brain and its extensive interconnectivity network running throughout the body (what they call the brain's *body-mapping system*). They, too, comprehend that mind/brain and body are inseparable.

Though the two books vary in approach, we find that each, in its unique way, reinforces the truth of Old Testament proverbial wisdom.

CASE PRESENTATION

J.M. is a twenty-two-year-old woman who was concerned about an abdominal sensation she had after eating. While she did not describe the problem as painful, she did say that she could "feel" the food moving through her intestine until well after it had been digested. She was worried that this might be abnormal. She also reported having, from time to time, a "tight feeling" in her neck and upper back. She didn't consider this painful, either, but she wondered about what she was experiencing.

Her medical tests were normal.

WHY YOU NEED TO LEARN A LITTLE NEUROBIOLOGY AND PHYSIOLOGY

Like the patient in the case above, you, too, may wonder what is going on inside your body. Understandably, you may also feel you can't describe it because you don't speak the doctor's language. When he or she uses those big, long, medical terms, your eyes glaze over. You're lost, except for mind-wandering recall of those science class lectures you nodded off in long ago. All of medicine's Latin and Greek-rooted words give you a headache.

The very title of this subsection may make you want to skip ahead. Don't.

The following scientific material is about structure and function—your structure and how you function. It's about the cells, nerves, genes, systems and interconnected relationships that make up you. Don't skip it. Take your time and plunge ahead.

You need to understand biologically how the mind/brain and body relate to and communicate with one another. Here are four good reasons why.

First, you know from your reading and personal experience that *somehow* your symptoms have emerged because living your life is hard, too fast-paced, complex, and very stressful. You weren't designed to live this way. *Somehow*, you have to look behind those symptoms to figure out what's really going on; and when you look at yourself (inside and out), you ought to know what you're looking at.

Second, you need to learn *how* and *why* symptoms develop if you are going to contend with each *somehow* described above.

Third, you'll first need some basic knowledge of the way your mind/brain and body systems are mapped out to function normally in balance and harmony with one another. (**PART 2**)

Fourth, you can then begin to appreciate how symptoms and disease arise when these same systems become imbalanced and inharmonious, resulting in dysfunction. (**PART 3**)

With the material from this chapter in hand, you will have the biological piece to your symptoms puzzle. Additionally, you will be able to reflect not only upon the psychological, social, and spiritual factors associated with not feeling like yourself, but comprehend as well their impact upon your biological make-up.

From this perspective, you will see that your symptoms embrace all elements of your being. They can't be evaluated part by part because your whole self is involved in their emergence. Knowing this, you will have the ability to look at yourself and look behind your symptoms to discover what they mean.

Your reflection on the why questions that lie behind and underneath your symptoms will prepare you for **PART 4** of the book. There you will be equipped with various tools that, as you grasp and use them, will assist you in finding health. The validation of your symptoms ordeal, through your own learning and by us, will be empowering. After you finish the book, you will be able to see a much bigger picture regarding your symptoms. You will no longer be overwhelmed by them. You will be the facilitator of your own self-care, interested in and able to absorb the emerging scientific findings that will complement your own self-discovery.

A CAVEAT: THEN CONTINUE READING

Your self-discovery must be ongoing.

Personal health is a life-long learning process.

HOW YOU EMERGE: A PRIMER ON YOUR BIOLOGICAL STRUCTURE AND FUNCTION

The focus of this chapter is the internal environment of your mind/brain and body. The external environment will be introduced in the next chapter. Knowing a little about the anatomy (structure) and physiology (function) of your internal environment will help you understand how YOU emerge. Like the place where you live, which was built from the ground up, we will look at the way you are put together by starting with the basic building block, the cell.

THE MICROSCOPIC COMMUNICATION SYSTEM OF CELLS AND CHEMICAL MESSENGERS

The first of four communication systems between the mind/brain and body is a low-level information transfer system operating at the level of the cells. You can't see the cells of the body and mind/brain or the chemicals that transfer information from cell to cell because they are microscopic.

Each cell is a small complex adaptive system and a building block of life.

The average adult human body contains an estimated one hundred trillion cells (counting one cell per second, it would take thousands of years to reach one hundred trillion). Despite the vast number of cells, an individual cell is invisible unless viewed under a microscope. The largest human cell is a female egg cell, which is approximately the diameter of a human hair. The smallest cell is the male sperm cell, which is one-tenth of the diameter of a human hair. Although the cells of your organ systems differ in size, shape, and function, all cells share key characteristics.

Each cell has several component parts. Particularly important to internal systems communication and function are the cell membrane and nucleus.

Every cell of your mind/brain and body must be able to relate and communicate with other cells. Here's how this happens.

The cell membrane surrounds each cell and serves as its doorway. On this outer surface are thousands of locations called *receptor sites*. Each receptor site functions as a lock capable of receiving a particular type of chemical messenger key, which floats in the fluid (*extracellular fluid*) surrounding each cell.

Dr. Candace Pert helped open the door to understanding receptors and the chemical messenger system. In *Molecules of Emotion: Why You Feel the Way You Feel*, she says: "If you were to assign a different color to each of the receptors that scientists have identified, the average cell surface would appear as a multicolored mosaic of at least seventy different hues—50,000 of one type of receptor, 10,000 of another, 100,000 of a third, and so forth."

The receptor lock in the cell membrane opens only by the insertion (*binding*) of a particular chemical messenger (*ligand*) floating in the extracellular fluid surrounding the cell. Chemical messenger keys can be *neuropeptides* (such as *enkephalin* or *endorphin*); *neurotransmitters* (such as *serotonin, norepinephrine,* and *acetylcholine*); and *steroids* (such as *estrogen* and *testosterone*). These chemical messenger keys insert themselves into the receptor keyholes.

A receptor lock is a single molecule, the smallest piece of a substance that can still be identified as that substance. The keyholes are actually vibrating in constant motion, serving as sensors or scanners waiting for a correct key chemical messenger. The receptor locks await the right chemical messenger keys to swim up to them through the extracellular fluid and to insert into the keyholes. While a key fitting into a lock is the common image, Dr. Pert says that a more dynamic description is to picture two voices, the chemical messenger key and the receptor lock, "striking the same note and producing a vibration that rings a doorbell to open the doorway to the cell."

Once within the keyhole, the key creates, as Dr. Pert describes it, "a disturbance to tickle the molecule into rearranging itself, changing its shape until – click! – information enters the cell." Now comes the amazing part. Having received the message from the chemical messenger key, the receptor lock transmits the information from the cell membrane to deep within the cell, where physiologic function can be dramatically changed. Examples of change in function include manufacturing new proteins, making decisions about cell division, and opening or closing tiny channels in the cell membrane, allowing electrolytes like sodium and potassium to enter and/or leave the cell. Thus, the function of a cell at any given moment is dependent upon which receptors are on its surface and whether chemical messengers occupy those receptors or not.

The keys themselves function in two different ways. They are either *agonists* or *antagonists*. As an agonist, the key fits into the lock and promotes a receptor mediated cellular process, stimulating the specific physiologic action for which the receptor is responsible. When functioning as an antagonist, the key has the opposite effect, inhibiting a receptor mediated cellular process. When either an agonist or antagonist key is engaged within a lock, no other can enter the keyhole.

The cells of your nervous system are called *neurons*. Your brain has approximately one hundred billion (100,000,000,000) neurons, and each neuron makes approximately 1000 connections with other neurons. Neurons have specialized projections called *dendrites* and *axons*. Dendrites bring information to the neuron and axons take information away. Crossing connections called *synapses*, information from one neuron flows to another via chemical messengers and electrical impulses.

Dr. Pert describes how all the cells of the mind/brain and body form a vast system network, in which all types of information, including emotional, circulate. That's why she calls her book *Molecules of Emotion*. She titles Chapter 9, "The Psychosomatic Network: A Concluding Lecture."

In it, Dr. Pert's use of the term *psychosomatic* carries a positive connotation. She describes an integrated information network intended to link the internal environment of the mind/brain and body. This is far different from the negative sense in which the term has been used by people who pejoratively label symptoms as "all in your head." Recalling the quotes at the beginning of the chapter, you can tie them to Dr. Pert's networking system. Whether the imagery used is a network, a body-mapping system, or proverbial wisdom, source materials that range from new science to the Old Testament confirm:

Your mind/brain and body cannot be separated.

They are intricately interconnected. From your mind/brain to other body parts and systems, the cell network allows organs to affect one another. Messages (and symptoms) coming from one spot in your body can reach virtually any other part of your body. The existence of this communications network explains how what you think or feel can affect positively and negatively every organ. An argument with a loved one can trigger abdominal cramps, even as a hoped-for reconciliation reduces them. Furthermore, the networking system also works in reverse. Body pain can affect your mood, temperament, and behavior. Keep this in mind when, in **PART 3,** you read how your internal systems become imbalanced and dysfunctional. For now, let's return to the structural building block, the cell, and see what's inside.

THE CELL NUCLEUS AND YOUR GENETIC MAKEUP

With the exception of your red blood cells, all of your cells have a nucleus, which is a sphere-like structure that controls and regulates the cell. The nucleus contains your genetic material, which is comprised of chromosomes. When cells divide, chromosomes do so as well. This process of chromosomal division is called *mitosis*.

There are twenty-three paired sets of twenty-three chromosomes, or forty-six chromosomes in all.

The first twenty-two pairs of chromosomes are numbered in sequence from one to twenty-two, while the twenty-third set of chromosomes is known as the X and Y pair. The two chromosomes of each pair are identical, with the exception of X and Y. The Y chromosome is present only in males. The X chromosome determines femaleness when paired with another X. When stained under a microscope, chromosomes show bands of light and dark areas. Each of the chromosome types has a unique pattern of bands.

Chromosomes are organized structures of proteins and the molecule *DNA* (*deoxyribonucleic acid*). Each chromosome contains a single continuous piece of DNA that looks like a twisted ladder. It is also known as the *double helix*. The DNA molecule is made up of four smaller molecules known as *bases* (A, T, C, and G). Each rung of the DNA ladder consists of two bases. The DNA molecule follows certain rules. A always pairs up with T, and C always pairs up with G. The sides of the ladder consist of a string of sugar and phosphate molecules, to which the rungs containing the bases attach. Each sugar-phosphate-base combination is called a *nucleotide*. In every one of your one hundred trillion cells, the sequence of these four letters or bases is nearly identical.

This unique sequence of four letters or bases in DNA is the *human genome*, your genetic material.

DNA contains the biological and genetic instructions that control the day-to-day function of your cells. DNA is like a blueprint, containing the directions necessary to construct other components of cells, such as proteins and RNA (ribonucleic acid). The instructions are passed down to you through inheritance. Genes are the DNA segments within chromosomes that carry genetic information and control the transmission and expression of one or more traits. They direct your cells to create the proteins that run the biochemical reactions of your bodies. There are an estimated 70,000 genes within the genome.

ORGAN SYSTEMS EMERGE FROM CELLS

Up to this point, we have focused on cells, the building blocks of complex adaptive systems. All of your cells are similar because they share the chemical messenger system. But there are many different types of cells, which are the parts of higher-level organ systems. During the first month of embryonic development, cells begin to specialize because of DNA turning on and turning off different sections of the information it stores. The cells are exact copies of their parent cells, formed when their parent cells divided. Even though the DNA code of the cells is the same, each cell type has a specific function. Examples include the cube-like cells of the intestine, which absorb the nutrients from food; the long and narrow muscle cells designed to contract; and the branched neurons of the nervous system designed to send and receive electrochemical impulses.

There are multiple organ systems at work within you, all of which are in relationship with one another.

The main organ systems of your body include:

CIRCULATORY SYSTEM: heart, blood, blood vessels, and lymphatics

DIGESTIVE SYSTEM: esophagus, stomach, small intestine, and colon

ENDOCRINE SYSTEM: pituitary, thyroid, ovaries, and testes

IMMUNE SYSTEM: organs (including lymphatics and spleen), special cells, proteins, and tissues

INTEGUMENTARY SYSTEM: skin, hair, nails, and sweat glands

MUSCULAR SYSTEM: muscles

NERVOUS SYSTEM: brain, spinal cord, and nerves

REPRODUCTIVE SYSTEM: uterus, penis, ovaries, and testes

RESPIRATORY SYSTEM: nose, larynx, trachea, diaphragm, bronchi, and lungs

SKELETAL SYSTEM: bones, cartilage, and joints

URINARY SYSTEM: kidneys, ureters, urinary bladder, and urethra

THE ABCDS OF YOUR INTERNAL ENVIRONMENT

With basic cell structure fundamentals in hand, you are ready to learn the ABCDs of your internal environment. In two important scientific/medical articles published in *Psychosomatic Medicine* in 2009, Dr. Richard D. Lane of the University of Arizona and his coauthors provide a comprehensive review of neuroscience in psychosomatic medicine. In discussing "pathways from mind to body," the authors utilize the following "classification system for different levels of function":

A) Mental/psychological/behavioral states and traits

B) Brain

C) Information transfer systems (autonomic nervous system [ANS], endocrine, immune)

D) Body proper (end organ function and dysfunction)

They emphasize that psychosomatic medicine currently focuses on levels A, C, and D. They go on to propose, "It is our thesis that the mind (A) can influence the body (D) only through levels B and C."

In our words, the mind/brain affects the body through the systems that transfer information. For clarity and simplicity, we will use, but modify, this classification system, integrating (A) with (B) into A/B, or mind/brain.

Keep in mind the microscopic communication system operating at the *low level* of the cells and chemical messengers and the classification system shown above. Now take a look at the *high level* communication systems.

MIND/BRAIN-BODY COMMUNICATION SYSTEMS (C)

There are three high level information transfer systems (C). We will call them the three mind/brain–body communication systems:

1) Nervous system,
2) Endocrine system,
3) Immune system.

These high-level systems emerge from and balance upon the low-level microscopic communication system. While they bear significant interactive responsibility,

the mind/brain interacts with the body mostly outside your conscious awareness.

The interaction occurs through these three systems. This interaction is bidirectional: mind/brain to body and body to mind/brain. The nervous system, especially the autonomic nervous system, and endocrine systems are primarily responsible for control of the visceral organs and the maintenance of homeostasis.

1) THE NERVOUS SYSTEM

The nervous system is one of the major organ systems of the body. It is actually several systems within one. The two main parts of your nervous system are the central nervous system (the brain and spinal cord) and the peripheral nervous system. Remember, for the sake of simplicity, we do not distinguish between mind and brain, but refer to them collectively as mind/brain.

Central Nervous System

Like the whole of you, the mind/brain is itself more than the sum of its parts. The human brain is a three-pound, cantaloupe-sized organ with a multi-folded surface, which greatly increases its surface area. As you can imagine, the mind/brain is the most important complex adaptive system of your body. Within it are many complex adaptive subsystems. The spinal cord is a tubular bundle of nerves, an extension of the central nervous system. It is enclosed and protected by the bones of the vertebral column. The primary function of the spinal cord is to transmit neural inputs between the body and the mind/brain.

Peripheral Nervous System

The peripheral nervous system is subdivided into the somatic nervous system and the autonomic nervous system. There are three subsystems of the autonomic nervous system, which will be discussed later in the chapter. The peripheral nervous system is your environmental interface. It is the interface between the internal environment of your mind/brain and body and the external environment around you. It is also the interface of the body with the mind/brain. Here's how the interfaces work.

Somatic Nervous System

The somatic nervous system includes 1) the senses and 2) sensory nerves called *homeostatic afferent nerves.*

1) The Six Senses

The somatic branch receives stressor input information from the external environment through your body's six senses. Yes, we said six senses, and we are not alluding to any telepathic sixth sense you may possess.

The five classical sensory systems of the body are touch, taste, sight, smell, and hearing/balance.

If they are not impaired or damaged, they input information from the external environment to the peripheral nervous system and ultimately into the mind/brain. Not all of us are able to use them all, but we are aware of them.

There is, however, a sixth sense: the gastrointestinal tract, or gut.

It is no misnomer when you talk about having a gut instinct. You can sense things in there. This sensory organ system is over thirty feet long. Believe it or not, it has a total surface area of 5,250 square yards (the size of a football field). Contrast this to the surface area of the skin, which is only two square yards. Your gut's enormous surface area contains *villi*, which are tiny finger-like projections that protrude from the gut surface. The villi greatly increase the surface area of the gastrointestinal tract, allowing nutrients to be more efficiently absorbed into the blood stream. Before they are absorbed, the gut senses and reacts to their source. Do you ever get particular sensations when eating certain foods? That's your gastrointestinal tract talking. It is the largest sense organ you have!

Let's turn the discussion to another of the six senses—vision. When not impaired, your eyes are the part of the body most representative of your sense of sight. The somatic peripheral nervous system is responsible for seeing and detecting anything that may threaten you, including any multitude of *stressors*. Again note the use of the term *stressor*. You will understand stress in an entirely new way after you have completed the book. For now, recall that stressors are external environmental inputs that result in internal *stress responses*, which seek to maintain and/or restore your body's balance and stability. Within your internal environment, the somatic peripheral nervous system conveys the information it receives to the mind/brain of the central nervous system.

While the emphasis is on the input of stressor information, the output of the peripheral nervous system is just as important. Detecting a threat, its output enables you to flee or fight by activating and controlling your skeletal muscles and autonomic nervous system (discussed in the next section).

2) The Homeostatic Afferent Nerves

As you now know, the somatic peripheral nervous system is functioning—detecting and relaying information—at two environmental interfaces:

→ **the external environment**—between the social and physical world around you and the internal environment of the mind/brain and body; and
→ **the internal environment**—between the body and the central nervous system (spinal cord and mind/brain).

Here, the focus continues to be on the internal environment of your mind/brain and body. Let's look at how it processes sensory input. In the December 2006 edition of *Gastroenterology*, Dr. Mayer, whose quote introduces this chapter, his colleague Dr. Bruce Naliboff, and neuroscientist, Dr. A.D. (Bud) Craig, explain two important dimensions of the mind/brain – body connection: *homeostatic feelings* and *homeostatic emotions.*

Key components in the connection are *homeostatic afferent nerves,* the tiny nerves of the peripheral somatic nervous system that supply all of the tissues of the body and send information from them to the spinal cord and ultimately to the mind/brain. Every tissue of the body is supplied with homeostatic afferent nerves: the skin, muscles, bones, joints, teeth, and all of the internal (visceral) organs, such as the heart, digestive tract, and liver. These nerves end (terminate) in the spinal cord. The spinal cord then relays what we call the *body words* spoken by the body to the mind/brain. Bodily communication with the mind/ brain through *body words* is an important concept that will be emphasized later. Our view is that,

The mind/brain is informed of the status of the whole body by the *body words* spoken by its parts.

Introducing this concept now provides you with an early look at how your symptoms are generated and serves as an example of why you must understand certain neuroanatomic aspects of your body-mind/ brain relationship. After all, it is in the spinal cord where short circuits can occur resulting in chronic pain and symptoms. You will learn about this harmful short circuiting, called *neuroplasticity,* in **PART 3** (Chapter 14).

Autonomic Nervous System (ANS)

The autonomic nervous system controls the functions of the organs and organ systems of the body. It has the primary responsibility of regulating four vital signs: heart rate, respiratory rate, blood pressure, and temperature. Recall that there is a fifth vital sign: pain. You will soon learn that:

The autonomic nervous system can play a key role in the generation and maintenance of chronic pain and medically unexplained symptoms because it is one of the most influential complex adaptive systems of the mind/brain-body.

The term *autonomic* means that the system is decentralized. There is no part of the autonomic nervous system that is in charge. The vital signs and function of the organs and organ system are fine-tuned by the autonomic nervous system, which is responsible for constantly adapting the body to environmental changes, both internal and external. While the somatic part of the peripheral nervous system has charge of input (and also the output of controlling muscular function),

The autonomic nervous system has output responsibilities in regulating the internal environment of your body.

Associated with vital internal functions, it helps maintain internal balance and stability (*homeostasis*) by coordinating activities like digestion, respiration, blood circulation, excretion, and hormone secretion. Your autonomic nervous system is always working. Since it operates reflexively and under the radar of consciousness, you are usually unaware of its continuous operation. The autonomic nervous system includes centers in the spinal cord, brain stem, hypothalamus, and thalamus. These centers also receive input from the emotional and cognitive systems of the mind/ brain, which you will be learning about later in the book. It is because of these connections with the other mind/brain systems that the autonomic nervous system can serve as the main component of the stress response system.

The autonomic nervous system contains three subsystems:

→ The sympathetic nervous system,
→ The parasympathetic nervous system, and
→ The enteric nervous system, which controls the gastrointestinal tract.

The **sympathetic** branch of your autonomic nervous system originates in the spinal cord. It goes into action to prepare the body for physical or mental activity. In response to a stressor, the sympathetic nervous system orchestrates what you familiarly call the *fight-or-flight* response. It increases muscle blood flow and tension, dilates pupils, accelerates heart rate and respiration, and increases perspiration and arterial blood pressure. To conserve and concentrate energy, it slows down digestive activity.

The **parasympathetic** branch of your autonomic nervous system also originates in your spinal cord. Activation of the parasympathetic nervous system causes a general slowdown in your body's functions to conserve energy. This is the *relaxation response*. Whatever the sympathetic nervous system dilates or accelerates the parasympathetic nervous system contracts or slows down.

The third branch of the autonomic nervous system is called the **enteric nervous system**. Dr. Jack Wood, a physiologist at The Ohio State University, has dubbed the enteric nervous system the "little brain in the gut." Given its roots, it is an apt description. The enteric nervous system is derived from the same part of a growing embryo as the brain. It has more neurons than the brain and has all of the brain's neurotransmitters, including serotonin. Serotonin is one of the neurotransmitter keys often implicated in depression. Remarkably, ninety-five percent of the serotonin in your body is located in the gut. Only five percent is found in the brain. The common embryologic origin of both the mind/brain and the gut brain is a clue to why the digestive system is the source of symptoms like abdominal pain, bloating, diarrhea, and constipation. Furthermore, the term "gut feeling" reflects accurately the fact that the little brain in the gut has something to do with intuition, instinct, and decision-making.

Curious, isn't it, that physiology confirms what you've known and felt for years?

We will leave you with your gut instincts for a while and move on to the endocrine system.

2) THE ENDOCRINE SYSTEM

The endocrine system is the second of the three mind/brain-body communication systems. It is a major organ system. There are two-way interactions between the endocrine system and the central nervous system. Responses of the endocrine system act over longer periods than do those of the autonomic nervous system and affect all the tissues and organ systems of the body. For example, *cortisol* is a hormone made in the two adrenal glands of the endocrine system, which sit on top of the kidneys. In response to stress and negative emotional states (e.g., fear, anxiety, and anger), the mind/brain of the central nervous system sends a chemical messenger to the adrenal glands through the bloodstream that instructs the adrenal glands to make cortisol. Cortisol is essential for life; however, when levels are elevated for prolonged periods in response to stress and/or negative emotion, cortisol is potentially harmful, causing and contributing to disease and even death.

3) THE IMMUNE SYSTEM

The immune system is the third of three mind/brain-body communication systems and is also one of the major organ systems of the body. There are two-way interactions between the central nervous system and the immune system. The mind/brain regulates immune function through the autonomic nervous and endocrine systems. Stress can suppress the immune system through mind/brain responses to the external environment, and the immune function can be adversely altered by depression and heart disease.

Whether viewed independently or collectively, all three mind/brain-body communication systems reflect the integrated pathway network between the mind/brain and the body.

As you will come to see, both your body and mind/brain are involved when it comes to how and why you are symptomatic.

IT'S NOT ALL IN YOUR HEAD!

What's really important here is that science continues to confirm that mental states (A) are linked to the brain (B), information transfer systems (C), and the body proper or disease (D). Your health and symptoms reflect this reality. With a system understanding of the mind/brain-body connection, you have reframed your understanding of how biological, psychological, social, spiritual, and behavioral factors can promote health or disease. In **PART 4** of the book, you will learn how to be healthy.

Through the receiving and processing of environmental stressor inputs (external and internal) and your output responses, YOU emerge. You express yourself through your body, feelings, emotions, consciousness, cognition, and behaviors. Note that *body* is emphasized and listed first. Here's the reason.

Your body has a lot to do with processing all the input you receive and the output you generate.

You are about to discover that all of the *body words* that you generate affect and greatly influence your bodily sensations and your sense of balance. This is why *body words* are formally called *homeostatic feelings*. As you will see, these homeostatic feelings are a key to how your symptoms and real pain are generated.

Hopefully, you have learned by now that your symptoms are not all in your head. But your head matters.

Here's why. It is of primary importance that the mind/brain knows at all times what is happening throughout your body. Bodily information, those *homeostatic feelings/body words* must be transmitted to your mind/brain so that the appropriate emotional, cognitive, and behavioral responses to whatever you are experiencing emerge.

Body words (homeostatic feelings) include:

→ Temperature (cool or warm)   → Salt craving

→ Muscle ache

→ Air hunger

→ Taste

→ Hunger

→ Sleepiness

→ Pain

→ Visceral sensations (chest, belly/gut, bladder, pelvis)

→ Sensual touch

→ Itch

→ Thirst

Pay particular attention to the *body word*, pain.

As you will soon learn, pain is much more complex than you may have thought. For now, ask yourself the following question.

HOW DO YOU FEEL?

Recent research and new discoveries are providing answers. In multiple disciplines, scientific breakthroughs—including the ability to take images of a living human brain—are revolutionizing our understanding of the relationship between your health and your mind/brain, body, feelings, emotion, consciousness, cognition, and behavior. Figure 10.1 is our simplified graphic representation of the four major mind/brain systems involved with feeling/symptoms, stress, emotion, and consciousness/cognition. Refer to Figure 10.1 now in the **Illustrations** section. Note how the four mind/brain systems all interrelate and overlap. This will become very important later in the book. The BODY TALK system depicted on the right side of the figure is responsible for how you feel.

HOW YOU EMERGE: BODY TALK SYSTEM

Dr. Craig says,

"The sense of the physiological condition of the body is called *interoception*." We call it the BODY TALK system.

The *body words* (homeostatic feelings) spoken by the body must first be heard by the BODY TALK system of the mind/brain. Once interpreted by the system, they are expressed as what we call *body talk*. The technical term for *body talk* is *homeostatic emotions*, and as with *body words*, *body talk* is a major factor impacting not only your sense of balance and physical sensation, but also the generation of your symptoms. Here's our summary of this critically important concept.

The mind/brain is informed of the status of the whole body in real time by the *body words* spoken by its parts. Once interpreted and translated, *body talk* emerges, expressed as feelings, emotions, cognitions, and symptoms.

The official name of the BODY TALK system is *the homeostatic afferent processing network* (*HAPN),* which is described by Doctors Mayer, Naliboff, and Craig. Using a little neuroanatomy and physiology, let's break down the acronym HAPN:

H is for Homeostatic (responsible for your dynamic internal balance);

A is for Afferent (responsive to signals traveling toward the central nervous system);

P is for Processing (active, receptive, integrative, and responsive);

N stands for Network (synonymous with system).

The HAPN includes the following brain structures: the *insular cortex* (*anterior insula*), the *anterior cingulate cortex*, the *thalamus*, and the *parabrachial nucleus*. While the details of most of these neuroanatomic structures are not essential in your studies, the insular cortex and anterior cingulate cortex of the BODY TALK system will reappear later in the book. As the bodily sensation processing network, the BODY TALK system translates and responds to all the sensations—the *body words*—that are related to your health. The system internally represents the physiologic state of the body. Relative to the *how* and *why* of symptoms, the BODY TALK system is the key *how* component of your internal stability. We propose that:

The BODY TALK system is the critical intersection where stress, feeling, emotion, consciousness, and behavior come together and out of which good and bad health may emerge.

Here's *how* your feelings emerge.

HOW YOU EMERGE: HOW THE BODY TALK SYSTEM WORKS

The BODY TALK system is a complex adaptive system. Once the *body words* are received and interpreted by the BODY TALK system, three responsive outputs emerge, as illustrated by Figure 10.2 in the **Illustrations** section.

In the figure, you notice that the three emergent responsive outputs are shown in the gray rectangles on the right. The first is the *intensity* of the response. This is your perception of the severity of what you are experiencing (how loud the *body words* are). The second is how it *affects* you and your *motivation* for alleviating the condition (whether the *body words* are upsetting and you feel the need to stop hearing them). The third response involves the *autonomic nervous system* (your heart races and you feel sweaty and shaky). In summary, once interpreted by the BODY TALK system, the *body words* (homeostatic feelings) are expressed as *body talk* (homeostatic emotions).

Dr. Antonio Damasio is Professor of Psychology, Neuroscience, and Neurology at the University of Southern California. In a trilogy of books that begins with *Descartes' Error*, he lays out the neural basis that links feeling (and emotion) and body and mind/brain interrelationships. Building upon Dr. Damasio's work, Dr. Craig has shown that pain is a homeostatic emotion (*body talk*). He writes:

"Humans perceive feelings—such as pain—from the body that provide a sense of their physiological condition and underlies mood and emotional state."

Can you see that it's more than simply a feeling?

THE PROBLEM OF PAIN

Recall that we advised you that pain is much more complex than you probably thought. There are several reasons this is true.

First, pain is a *body word*/homeostatic feeling that must be heard, interpreted, and expressed as *body talk*/homeostatic emotion by the BODY TALK system. For example, if the BODY TALK system interprets and expresses pain as severe, causing you enough distress that you seek consultation and relief, and triggers associated unpleasant autonomic symptoms (e.g., racing heart, sweat, nausea), then you're sick. You're hurting with real disease.

Second, we have emphasized the interrelationships and overlaps among the four mind/brain systems. Suppose your thoughts are negative. What if you are also anxious and/or depressed? You're stressed out, too. All four mind/brain systems are at work here. The outcome is greater suffering and pain. Pain is complex and involves both the body and mind/brain. It's just not possible to separate them.

Third, if you are symptomatic, you might be asking yourself,

Why should I be hurting like this?

What have I done to be suffering so much?

Previously, we quoted C.S. Lewis:

"Pain hurts. That is what the word means."

If you are interested in reading Lewis further, he addresses pain and suffering in *The Problem of Pain* and *A Grief Observed*. We think his cited observation states a subtly obvious truth and submit that pain may call attention to and/or be exacerbated by the spiritual questions and issues he raises in his work. We will have more to say about this in Chapter 18.

FROM BODY WORDS TO TALK TO DIALOGUE

The BODY TALK system is crucially important in maintaining homeostasis of the interrelationships of the body with the mind/brain and for your survival.

When the BODY TALK system is functioning optimally, you are in balance and more likely to feel well. When dysfunction occurs in one or more of the three BODY TALK system responses, distressing symptoms may emerge, as you will come to understand in Chapter 14.

At this point, it is enough to understand how the functioning of the BODY TALK system helps explain the causal association of physical, emotional, and psychological symptoms with negative thinking, anxiety, depression, and stress. In our view,

The translation of *body words* into *body talk* provides the opportunity for true dialogue between body and mind/brain.

This will be a critical topic in **PART 3** of the book.

BODY MAPS IN YOUR BRAIN

By now, you should be getting a picture of the remarkable interrelationship between your body and your mind/brain. As you have learned, your mind/brain must know what is happening in your body at all times. Multiple body maps emerge within your mind/brain, which represent the real-time state of your body. Your mind/brain generates a road atlas of your body that is constantly updated. As described in *The Body Has a Mind of Its Own*, the Blakeslees show that just as road maps represent interconnections across the landscape, multiple body maps in your brain represent all aspects of your bodily self, inside and out. Your physical and emotional awareness and sense of being a whole, feeling person emerge from the complex interrelationships of the many body maps within your brain.

While mind/brain mapping occurs in mammals, the BODY TALK system is unique to primates and is most highly developed in humans.

So while your dog is an emotional animal, s/he just doesn't feel like you do!

I KNOW MY DOG HAS FEELINGS!

You're right. Your dog is an emotional animal, but s/he doesn't have the same connections between the body and the mind/brain. Your dog has feelings from the body, but there's no BODY TALK system to receive them. After reading Chapter 16 (The Emotions Are Embodied), you will see this clearly.

LINK

With most of your anatomy and physiology primer completed, you will now examine both the social and physical world in which you live and the impact of genetic makeup on personal health. Read on to learn how your health relates to and is affected by your external environment and heredity.

CHAPTER 11

How YOU Emerge: Balance, Heredity, and YOUR External Environment

QUESTION

How do heredity and the external environment relate to my health?

QUOTE

"Health depends on a state of equilibrium among the various factors that govern the operation of the body and the mind; equilibrium, in turn, is reached only when man lives in harmony with his external environment."

Treatise on Air, Water, and Places
HIPPOCRATES (known as "the father of Western medicine," 460-370 B.C.E.)

ABOUT THE QUOTE

Good health is not solely a matter of mind/brain/body equilibrium. As Hippocrates attests, it is also dependent upon a person being in harmony with the external environment. You are a product of nature and nurture. Necessarily, your mind and body must be in balance with the world around you. This is a dynamic, not static, enterprise. On this point, Albert Einstein offers apt advice. Comparing life to riding a bicycle, he says in a letter to his son,

"To keep your balance, you have to keep moving."

This is true, even when it hurts.

CASE PRESENTATION

T.J. is a fifty-five-year-old man who suffers from abdominal pain and headaches. In response to questions regarding the frequency and severity of his symptoms, he acknowledged that abdominal pain and headaches had bothered him on and off for many years, but had begun only recently to interfere with his daily life. He admitted having trouble sleeping, and he indicated that he felt fatigued much of the time. Lately, he said, his pain became worse in the afternoon while he was still at work. Asked whether his symptoms were related to any stress in his life, he disclosed that he did not get along well with his boss. The work environment was difficult and he said he felt considerably better on weekends. He also acknowledged that both the pain and headaches became worse when he and his wife weren't doing well. Last, he added that he had come to realize that his symptoms were more severe during winter or when there was a stretch of overcast, sunless weather. When asked about his family history, he recalled that his father had similar symptoms and suffered with depression.

All of his medical tests were normal.

HOW YOU EMERGE REVISITED

Chapter 10 focused upon the internal environment of your body. Now we turn to the external environment of the world in which you live. After you finish this chapter, you will see the big picture of how you emerge. YOU—your body, feelings, emotions, consciousness, cognition, memory, and behavior—emerge from both the external environment and the internal environment of your body and mind/brain. You emerge from both the nurture of the external environment and the nature of your internal environment, the latter of which is influenced by your genetics and gender.

TWO ENVIRONMENTS IN RELATIONSHIP

As T.J.'s case presentation suggests, there is more to being healthy or symptomatic than mere body chemistry. While T.J.'s medical tests revealed nothing that would explain his symptoms, his responses to the examination questions were revealing. Work stressed him. His marriage could stress him. Sunlight deprivation stressed him. He may have inherited vulnerability to stress-induced depression from his father. In relationship to various facets of his external environment, T.J. was disharmonious and out of balance.

Out of balance, he becomes diseased and symptomatic.

That he was symptomatic should come as no surprise. He did not live in an insulated cocoon. Neither do the rest of us. We each relate to and are a product of our environments and genetic heritage. In Chapters 9 and 10, you learned about the intricacies of the various systems of the mind/ brain and body. You learned that not only are you made up of a multitude of complex adaptive systems, you are one yourself. You are constantly connecting, reacting, and adapting to the world around you. Your internal environment and balance are interdependent and in dynamic relationship with the external environment.

THE BODY HAS A MIND OF ITS OWN

The last sentence of the previous paragraph may seem to state the obvious. Try reflecting on it from a fresh, neuroscientific research perspective. In the previous chapter, you learned about body maps in the brain described by Sandra Blakeslee and Matthew Blakeslee in *The Body has a Mind of Its Own*. In their introduction, they write:

Your self does not end where your flesh ends, but suffuses and blends with the world, including other beings. Thus, when you ride a horse with confidence and skill, your body maps and the horse's body maps are blended in shared space. When you make love, your body maps and your lover's body maps commingle in mutual passion.

This is a remarkable quote. When you think about being in touch with what's around you, you see that the passage gives new meaning to the relationship between personal space and external connection. The point, of course—whether it is obvious or fresh—is that you and your external environment are intricately related. The connection is so critical that your health and well-being depend upon cultivating harmony between you and your world. Harmonizing yourself with the environment is tricky business, especially when you take into account the matter of heredity. This is a fact for you and the federal government. In a September 4, 2007 news release issued by the National Institute of Health, Mike Leavitt, then Secretary of the Department of Health and Human Services, states:

"Researchers have long known that our genes, our environmental exposures and our behavioral choices all have an influence on our health."

The quote succinctly summarizes the position statement of the National Institute of Environmental Health Sciences (NIEHS), which is part of the National Institutes of Health. On its web site, the NIEHS declares:

Almost all diseases are related to complex interaction between an individual's genetic make-up and environmental agents. Subtle differences in genetic factors cause people to respond differently to the same environmental exposure. This explains why some individuals have a fairly low risk of developing a disease resulting from an environmental insult, while others are much more vulnerable. As scientists learn more about how genetics and environmental factors work together to cause human diseases, they will be able to develop new strategies for the prevention and treatment of many diseases. The Genes and Environment Initiative is a five-year, NIH-wide effort to identify the genetic and environmental basis of asthma, diabetes, cancer, and other common illnesses. This initiative will support the development of new procedures for analyzing genetic variation in groups of patients with specific illnesses, and new technologies for measuring exposures to chemical and biological agents, dietary intake, physical activity, psychosocial stress, and addictive substances.

This complex interaction between your genetic make-up and the environment demands closer scrutiny.

A simplified composite of the world around you consists of:

1. the natural physical;
2. the man-made physical; and
3. the social (individual activity and interpersonal interaction).

For ease of reference, we will stick to these three components when discussing the external environment. They are common sense. While we are aware of how treacherous it has become to navigate a course between environment and health (the impact of diet, pollutants, toxins, weather, and climate change comes to mind),

We believe the genetics and environment interface factor really makes clear sailing difficult.

Why is this? First, we often see and feel the effects of genetics and environment upon our health. Suppose your mother suffered from chronic headaches. Not only might you be genetically predisposed to have the same symptom, you may have also learned to express stress through the symptom of headache. Perhaps you weren't treated well when you were growing up. Maybe you're constantly stressed by a difficult relationship with a loved one or coworker. Like genetic vulnerability factors, aversive life events (especially physical, emotional, and/or sexual abuse occurring during infancy and childhood) are life-long environmental vulnerability influences. In medical parlance, these aversive life events are called *epigenetic*. In biology, the term refers to changes in gene expression.

Second, interactions between the *dis-ease* you may feel (symptoms) and environmental stressors are bi-directional. While environmental factors determine whether genes are turned on and expressed, genetic variability influences the way you respond symptomatically to your environment by influencing organ systems, particularly the central nervous system. Inherited interacting genetic variants affect molecular alterations at the cellular level and ultimately influence organ systems. Within the organ system of the central nervous system, they predispose and bias interactions, interrelationships, information processing, and *neuroplasticity* (the capacity for the mind/brain to change in structure, organization, and function). This results in your symptoms and ultimately affects your behavior. These variants are another wild card in multidimensional health care models.

Recall the weaknesses of the biopsychosocial model. Here's another important one. Joel Paris, M.D., is a professor of psychiatry at McGill University. In *Nature and Nurture in Psychiatry,* he writes:

The biopsychosocial model has been helpful in encouraging psychiatrists to think multidimensionally. However, it has one serious defect: it fails to explain why some individuals develop one category of mental disorder while other individuals develop a completely different category of illness. This question can only be addressed by assuming that individual differences in susceptibility to mental disorders are rooted in biological vulnerability.

Your inherited susceptibilities to environmental influences are important.

TEMPERAMENT AND VULNERABILITY

Temperament and vulnerability are inherited predispositions to environmental influences. They are necessary, but not alone sufficient for the development of mental disorders. Necessary conditions are those that must be present for a disorder to develop. Sufficient conditions are those in whose presence a disorder will inevitably develop. Predisposing genetic conditions also affect behaviors, which can be harmful or helpful to health.

Environmental factors determine whether genetic predispositions cross a threshold of vulnerability and develop into disorders.

Stressors by themselves are rarely sufficient environmental influences for the development of mental disorders. Resilience is the rule rather than the exception, and most people go through life carrying predispositions to psychopathology that are never expressed. Usually, only severe and repeated stressors uncover these vulnerabilities. Single events often cause short-term symptoms, but rarely lead to lasting psychopathology.

Let's expand this concept to *dis-ease* and symptoms. Dr. Paris also writes,

"At the interface of psychiatry and medicine, we can apply the same model to 'psychosomatic disorders'."

As you now know, this pejorative term is often used in reference to medically unexplained functional symptoms and syndromes. When used pejoratively, psychosomatic implies that the illness is all in one's head. However, the interaction of genetics and environment affects not only the mind/brain, but also the mind/brain–body relationship and helps explain medically unexplained symptoms and symptom syndromes (functional somatic syndromes). Gastroenterologist Emeran Mayer's quote introduced Chapter 9. As an editor of the medical journal *Gastroenterology*, he says in an article in the June 2008 issue, "The Challenge of Studying the Biology of Complex, Symptom-Based GI Disorders":

Like other complex, symptom-based disorders, it is expected that functional gastrointestinal disorders are caused by numerous genetic and environmental factors, each of which has individually small effects, and that only result in full disease expression in a given individual if their combined effects cross a 'threshold of liability.'

What does this mean for you?

CROSSING THE THRESHOLD OF LIABILITY

Dr. Mayer refers to another term that is familiar to you: *comorbidity* (the association and coexistence of symptoms, including such symptoms as anxiety, fatigue, non-gastrointestinal pain conditions, and somatization). He writes,

Not surprisingly, the same mistake has been made by many fields outside gastroenterology (including rheumatology and urology), where specific organ-based symptom criteria (for fibromyalgia or interstitial cystitis) have been established, under the exclusion of frequently 'comorbid' GI or psychiatric symptoms.

In summary, our point is that,

Dis-ease, including medically unexplained symptoms and functional somatic syndromes, is related to both nature and nurture.

T.J.'s father had symptoms similar to his own. Nature versus nurture is not an either/or question. Each plays a pivotal role in how you emerge. The real issue is not a simplistic choice of one factor over the other. Your life is more complex than that. The pivotal question is how the interaction between your genetic makeup and the environment can shift the balance between heath and disease. It is a question of complexity and balance.

Think about what you already know about genetics, not simply from the Chapter 10 primer, but from your own experience. Certain family traits may come to mind. Perhaps it's the shape of your nose, your hair color, skin sensitivity, or the size of your ears. If family members in previous generations (parents/grandparents) share characteristics you possess, you probably inherited the trait. The term *heredity* signifies this transmission of genetic traits from parents to offspring. In some families, the trait is a source of pride or stature. Perhaps it's a strong chin, eye color, or musculature. In others, an inherited trait may be the butt or bane of family lore.

Regardless of how you appraise inherited characteristics, you are a product of your genes. They shape and regulate not only how you look, but also how you process the world around you.

As you'll remember from Chapter 10, your genes are paired on chemical strands known as DNA. DNA is stored in each cell of your body. The genes' source was the sperm and egg from which you came. Through repeated cell division, skin, bones, brain tissue, and muscle were formed. Directed by your genes, the cells connected to one another to make you YOU. In the 100 trillion-plus cells of which you're made, each contains a copy of that first pair of genes. Their make-up actively determines development throughout your life. If you have children, you pass them on, though not exactly in the same configuration each time. If you have more than one child, you've probably commented about their sharing similar traits, yet each being unique. The gene blend is slightly different each time a sperm and egg unite.

During the process of the cell's division, additional variation can occur. Recall that your genes' directives are set forth in a four-letter chemical code known as ATG and C. The sequences of the chemicals dictate to the genes how to manufacture the protein that will affect the genes' directives. As the code is transcribed throughout cell division, errors can and do take place. Some are serious. Disease can be inherited (such as sickle cell anemia), the result of one letter of the ATG and C code having been miscopied along the way.

However, regarding the complex interaction between genetic make-up, environment, and your health, most disease is not the consequence of one miscopied gene acting by itself, but the result of its interaction with some provoking element in the environment.

The provoking element might be natural, man-made, or social. It could be a food substance, industrial pollution, or behavioral choice, like smoking.

LIFE'S COMPLEXITIES

Recall the word *genome* from Chapter 10, which is the set of genes that governs the workings of every human cell. In an article entitled "Life's Complexities," in the July 13, 2009 issue of *Newsweek*, Fred Guteri points out that only a little more than one percent of the genome consists of genes that produce the proteins responsible for running the cell's operations. The exact role of the other ninety-nine percent is not yet clear, but we do know that only a few diseases are caused by a single gene. Some originate from a variety of subsets containing tens of thousands of genes. To add further to the complexities of life, health, and disease, the packing of genes in the cell may have as much to do with development and disease as the genes themselves. This packing arrangement, *epigenetics*, may even account for inherited traits passed on to generations.

Epigenetics is essentially inheritance without DNA and this discovery is leading to remarkable scientific progress regarding understanding and treating disease.

Guteri goes on to declare,

"The realization that the cell is a complex entity greater than the sum of its parts has forced doctors on the forefront of medical research to consider their patients as biological 'systems.' This awareness is now transforming the way medicine is practiced and taught."

Here's another layer of complexity.

There is considerable variability in the genome in what is known as copy number variation (CNV), which is actually very common in everybody's genome.

These are duplications or deletions of segments of a chromosome, which involve combinations of genes that depress or enhance the actions of specific genes. One example of a CNV is an extra copy of chromosome twenty-one that results in Down syndrome. One specific type of CNV is called *de novo* mutations. It occurs in only one bodily tissue—the sperm or egg—and may crop up relatively late in life during reproduction and appear only in the next generation. As Nobel Prize winner, Dr. Eric Kandel, describes in the same issue of *Newsweek*, this fits the pattern of autism, which is a genetic disease that occasionally emerges in families in which healthy parents who are free of autism pass the disorder down to one of their children even though the mutation does not appear in their chromosomes, but only in their sperm or eggs. The autistic child could pass the mutation on from generation to generation.

EXAMPLES OF BOTH NATURE AND NURTURE

From your learning, you are going to apply your knowledge to understanding more fully how you emerge in relationship to nature and nurture. Recall the mind/brain-body communication systems described in Chapter 10. There serotonin was considered to be one of the important chemical messengers in the brain and body (particularly in the digestive tract). A recent article by S.F. Dingfelder in *Monitor on Psychology* describes how a certain gene gives instructions to produce a molecule that moves serotonin out of the synapse. A short variant of the gene increases the rate of production of the molecule, causing serotonin to move too quickly. Because serotonin may play a role in the cause of depression, having this vulnerability gene variant might result in symptoms of depression, but this variant vulnerability gene is common, and most who have it don't suffer with depression.

Another influencing factor is the external environment. Both nature and nurture impact and are impacted by it. Vulnerabilities may arise. For example, having the variant gene may increase sensitivity to the environment. Moreover,

If the environment was or is challenging (e.g., early life abuse, stress, poverty), then the symptoms of depression may emerge as a reflection of the combination of nature and nurture.

Let's decipher this further. As you now know, there is a relationship between life stress and depression. Why does stress lead to depression in some people but not in others? Those who are vulnerable to depression may differ in the make-up of a gene called the *serotonin transporter gene*. Those with a short form of a specific section of the gene are at greater risk for depression. Extending this remarkable scientific understanding,

New research confirms that depression patients' brain circuitry makes them vulnerable to relapse.

Using brain imaging that assesses for dysfunction with positron emission tomography (PET), National Institute of Mental Health researchers, led by Doctors Wayne Drevets and Gregor Hasler, have produced direct evidence that:

People prone to depression—even when they're feeling well—may have abnormal mood-regulating brain circuitry.

This makes them vulnerable to relapse when levels of certain key brain chemical messengers plummet. Indirect evidence had previously suggested that people with histories of depression had such an abnormality in the brain systems that communicate by using the chemicals dopamine and norepinephrine. Dopamine normally inhibits runaway activity of emotion hubs deep in the brain. Depleting dopamine effectively takes the brakes off the emotional hubs in depression-prone individuals, thereby increasing circuit activity and vulnerability to relapse.

Recent research addresses the role of nature/genetic and nurture/environmental factors in the etiopathogenesis (read: cause) of fibromyalgia syndrome (FMS) and other related symptom syndromes (functional somatic syndromes), such as irritable bowel syndrome.

Studies confirm that there is a high aggregation of fibromyalgia in families of fibromyalgia patients. First-degree biological relatives of individuals with fibromyalgia have an 8-fold greater risk of developing fibromyalgia compared with the general population. Family members of individuals with irritable bowel syndrome have almost three times the odds of developing irritable bowel syndrome. The mode of inheritance is unknown, but it is probably *polygenic*, which means it involves multiple genes. There is evidence that *polymorphisms*, or alterations in genes involved with certain chemical messengers, such as *serotonin*, *dopamine*, and *catecholamines*, play a role in the etiology of fibromyalgia. These polymorphisms are not specific for FMS and are associated with other functional somatic disorders, anxiety, and depression.

WHAT DETERMINES WHICH SYMPTOMS ARE EXPRESSED?

Genetic predispositions of temperament and vulnerability influence the specific symptoms that are expressed. In the same way that a gene in a vulnerable relationship with the environment can play a role in the expression of the symptoms of depression, a similar vulnerability gene or combination of genes could result in the expression of symptoms in any bodily system.

The potential impact of both genetic and environmental influences on the four mind/brain systems may trigger:

→ **enhanced pain sensitivity in any bodily system, distress, and autonomic response** (BODY TALK System)
→ **increased stress reactivity** (STRESS RESPONSE System)
→ **depressed mood and/or anxiety** (EMOTIONAL System)
→ **negative thoughts** (CONSCIOUSNESS System)

Dr. Mayer references cognitive neuroscientist Dr. Tyrone Cannon, also from UCLA, and suggests that complex, symptom-based disorders (such as irritable bowel syndrome and fibromyalgia) are caused by numerous genetic and environmental factors, each of which has individually small effect, and results in full disease expression in a given individual only if their combined effects cross the threshold of liability. For example, despite the presence of vulnerability genes, the threshold for irritable bowel syndrome might not be crossed if the necessary environmental co-factors (such as irritation of the digestive tract by certain foods or infection) are not present. The same vulnerability genes may result in the expression of a different functional somatic syndrome like fibromyalgia, or in a psychiatric syndrome, such as depression.

Recognizing the complexity of genetic/environmental interrelationships helps to explain the presence of multiple symptoms and the overlap of symptoms and functional somatic syndromes.

You have already learned of the symptom association of irritable bowel syndrome and fibromyalgia. In explaining the overlap, consider how each of us may adopt different behavioral strategies to cope with stress, based upon different genetically determined personalities and physiological response tendencies.

Doctors Korte, Koolhaas, Wingfield, and McEwen write that, from an evolutionary perspective, there are both males and females with high aggression (Hawks) personality types who tend to respond behaviorally with fight-flight. Others, with low aggression (Doves) personalities, tend to express freeze-hide behavioral responses.

Thus, good stress adaptive processes that actively maintain stability through change (allostasis) depend in part on the personality types and their associated stress responses. The benefits of allostasis and the costs of bad stress adaptation (allostatic load) lead to different trade-offs in health and disease.

Collectively, this provides some explanation of why individuals may differ in their vulnerability to different stress-related diseases. Among personality types, Hawks—due to inefficient management of chemical messengers of allostasis—are more likely to be violent, to develop impulse control disorders, hypertension, cardiac arrhythmias, sudden death, atypical depression, chronic fatigue states, and inflammation. In contrast, Doves, due to the greater release of chemical messengers of allostasis (surplus), are more susceptible to anxiety disorders, metabolic syndromes, melancholic depression, psychotic states, and infection. Personality type is but one factor involved.

Gender also matters. Gender has a strong influence on bodily symptom reporting.

Dr. Kroenke confirms that physical symptoms that are presented for primary care are fifty percent or more likely to be reported by women than by men. One important factor is an increased prevalence of depression, anxiety, and somatoform disorders in women. However, a complex variety of environmental, biological, genetic, and gender factors are involved. Fortunately, it's unlikely to be quite as far out as being from different planets as John Gray suggests in his book title, *Men Are from Mars, Women Are from Venus*, but gender does matter when it comes to symptoms.

YOU ARE UNIQUELY COMPLEX

What makes the specific interaction between gene make-up and environmental elements problematic is that not everyone suffers similar consequences. You probably know someone who has smoked cigars all his life and is hale and hearty at age ninety-two. Sadly, you've likely known someone else who never smoked a day in her life and yet died of lung cancer when she was sixty-one. How do you account for the differences? This is a cutting edge question for researchers as they investigate how and why people react in different ways to elements in the environment.

If you reread the website declaration of the NIEHS, which we cited earlier, you can sense not only growing awareness, but also keen investigative interest in deciphering the variability of human reaction to environmental elements.

Already, researchers have begun making progress in identifying genes that appear to influence the ways in which you might react. What scientists have learned is not that such genes cause your disease, but that they may predispose you to be more susceptible to having an adverse reaction from exposure. Some of you may have a gene variation that increases risks associated with radiation exposure. Others may have a gene characteristic that is more resistant to similar exposure. Study and research continue in the hope that you and your doctor may someday be able to identify and discuss all the environmental elements you might not be resistant to and therefore need to avoid.

Sorting out what's important regarding environmental influences on your health isn't easy.

In his book, *Hyping Health Risks*, epidemiologist Geoffrey Kabat describes how activists, regulators, and scientists can distort or magnify tiny environmental risks, inflating small findings into dubious claims. He is concerned about how "the highly charged climate surrounding environmental health risks can create powerful pressure for scientists to conform and to fall into line with a particular position."The risk is that linear thinking will reduce appreciation of non-linear complexity.

What's important is that you know that you are a complex being living in a complex, nonlinear world.

No wonder everyone's vision is blurry.

CAN YOU SEE THE BIG PICTURE?

Can you see that a focus on symptoms alone is an exercise in futility? Can you see that linear thinking that tries to carefully classify symptoms into syndromes, distinguish symptoms as either organic or functional, and then apply diagnostic labels to symptom collections is incompatible with seeing the true complexity that is involved?

The whole is greater than the sum of its parts.

Focusing on the symptoms distracts you from asking the critical question,

What's behind the symptoms?

By asking, you can be an active participant in your own self-care. You are probably already aware of environmental elements to which you react. They may be certain foods, allergens, or the sun. These are common. You may also be susceptible to other elements in the environment that are unique to you and your family tree.

Therefore, it is important to learn as much family health and medical history as you can. You will learn how to do this in PART 4.

Pass the information down. Seek out the family medical history before there's no one left who can share it with you. There may be family susceptibilities, tendencies, or predispositions, the knowledge of which is vital to your health. Become self-educated and aware. If there have been family members who seemed prone to excessive drinking, bouts of despondency and dejection, or extreme anxiety or worry, learn their life stories. Read up on scientific and medical inquiry into genetic susceptibility and predisposition. The more awareness you gain, the better able you will be to identify your family history when you fill out those medical forms. It's tedious, but it may contain a clue to why you hurt.

THE WISDOM BEHIND THE SYMPTOM

We counsel you to use your hurt to ask what's behind the symptoms and reflect on your life. Learn your genetic history as best you can. Don't leave your pain to others to decipher. It's not all in your head, as some would superficially surmise. Yet in dealing with what's wrong, your mind/brain is part of the problem. It can also be critical to your healing.

Your mind/brain is plastic, flexible, and capable of remapping a way out of the hurt.

As you question and reflect, ponder these words of Justice Felix Frankfurter as well:

"Wisdom too often never comes, and so one ought not to reject it merely because it comes late."

It's not too late to learn; and your brain is never too old to rethink, adapt, and change. Even if your pain seems endless, it is never too late, not simply to make life endurable, but to imagine yourself well.

Unlearning and reframing your understanding of your *dis-ease* and symptoms are as important, if not more so, than taking medication.

In a scientific study, headed by Dr. Tomas Furmark of Uppsala University in Uppsala, Sweden, patients with social phobia were treated for several weeks, using either cognitive behavioral therapy or an antidepressant drug called *citalopram*. They were then brain-scanned while speaking in public. The study showed that symptoms improved significantly and about equally with either CBT or antidepressant drug therapy with citalopram. In functional brain images, CBT and the drug had similar effects on the emotional brain center, including the amygdala. The study reinforces the value of learning to look at your symptoms from a different angle because reframing your understanding is a key to finding health. One of the available reframing resources may come as a surprise to you.

LINK

As you will read in Chapter 12, it is the imagination—as much as it is knowledge—that is instrumental in self-discovery and renewal.

CHAPTER 12

YOUR Health and the Inner Life Tie That Binds

QUESTION

Can I imagine myself well?

QUOTES

Tradition teaches that soul lies midway between understanding and unconsciousness, and that its instrument is neither the mind nor the body, but imagination. I understand therapy as nothing more than bringing imagination to areas that are devoid of it, which then must express themselves by becoming symptomatic.

Care of the Soul, xiii
THOMAS MOORE

"Imagination is more important than knowledge. For while knowledge defines all we currently know and understand, imagination points to all we might yet discover and create."

"What Life Means to Einstein," *The Saturday Evening Post*, vol. 202, October 26, 1929
ALBERT EINSTEIN

Imagining is perhaps as close as humans get to creating something out of nothing the way God is said to. It is a power that to one degree or another everybody has or can develop, like whistling. Like muscles, it can be strength-

ened through practice and exercise. Keep at it until you can actually hear your grandfather's voice...

Whistling in the Dark
FREDERICK BUECHNER

ABOUT THE QUOTES

Despite new research that indicates the presence of the brain's intricate body-mapping systems, and despite the revival of interest in holistic health care practices of ancient healing traditions, many care practitioners continue to cling to dualistic concepts that separate mind and body. As we have pointed out, this tendency remains prevalent regardless of its diagnostic limitations, including the inability to account for illness without disease. From the outset, we have lamented the practice of splitting patients and other care recipients into segregated segments and treating them part by part. Although care models built on mind/body dualism do not easily give way to cutting edge research or wisdom recovered from the past, there is hope that health care practitioners may once again ground themselves in an integrated, holistic understanding of their patients. Part of the reason for hope rests in you.

Your personal reorientation to imagining your own well-being is a key to your becoming your own health care advocate.

Previously, you've read about the intricate systemic linkage between your mind/brain and body. You've studied and reflected upon the importance of harmonious relationship between your internal and external environments. These are lessons vital to balance and self-understanding. There is another facet integral to linked and balanced relationships that we have alluded to but not yet fully discussed. It isn't additional knowledge or greater conscious thought because, as you know from experience, thinking by itself is often part of the symptomatic problem. The more you think and dwell upon a problem, the worse it often seems to become. This is true, even though the vast majority of what you fret over and worry about never materializes.

Nor is it stepping up to embody a single-minded commitment to a physical regimen. Your body, however fit, if otherwise lacking perceptual and emotional stability, can produce bad stress responses (allostatic load) to the stressors you experience. This is one of the reasons you may become symptomatic.

Given these self-limiting constraints, there must be another facet to your makeup, something integral to helping harmonize your whole being, internally and externally.

Necessarily, it must be intimately familiar with your mind/brain and body, but not held captive by either. Because your well-being is a matter of both the homeostatic balance of your internal environment and your being in harmony with the external environment, it must be able to embrace each environment and serve as bridge between them.

What is this something?

What helps give harmony, balance, and inspiration to the physical, emotional, mental, spiritual, interpersonal, social, cultural, natural, environmental, and cosmic aspects of your being? Imagine for a moment what it might be. This question and our response are the subjects of this chapter.

CASE PRESENTATION

In 2003, doctors diagnosed C.H. with a brain tumor. Earlier symptoms had indicated progressive hearing loss and physical balance issues, not the kind of problems easily dealt with while teaching high school freshman. C.H. met with her doctor, underwent further tests, and then consulted with an otolaryngologist, neurologist, and neurosurgeon.

During consultation, C.H. learned that she had two surgical options. The surgeons could go after the tumor through the back of her head. This was the higher-risk approach, given the intricate volume of brain cells they would have to cut around. The second option was to enter from the side near the ear. This was less risky, but guaranteed right-side hearing loss. C.H. listened, asked questions, and weighed the risks. By nature and attitude, C.H. is hopeful, plucky, optimistic, and resolute. She is expressive and spiritually grounded. Nevertheless, choosing between high risk and specific loss was difficult and further complicated by her medical history.

In early elementary school, C.H. began blacking out. Falling off a teeter-totter or swing set became the norm. When she hit the ground, she could not move or otherwise respond to worried siblings and friends. C. H. was diagnosed with epilepsy. Medication and a watchful family kept physical harm in check. Still on medication and at risk for blacking out, she started high school, but always the cheerful, bright-side optimist, she imagined well the four years to come.

During her freshman year, C.H. contracted encephalitis, a severe inflammation of the brain. For days, she was in a coma. Her family, friends, and an aging minister prayed and kept vigil by her bed. Critically ill, comatose, C.H. was touch and go. Eventually, she regained consciousness. Her recovery was slow; she was months behind in school.

There were other consequences. Given the trauma to the brain, C.H. lost her sense of smell and suffered nerve damage that affected her hands. She had to re-learn how to write. Through her coma, recovery, and guarded care, family and sibling dynamics took on new forms. Roles and relationships were reshaped. In light of her medical history, having to face surgery forty years later was an exceptionally difficult prospect. C.H.'s brain and the rest of her nervous system had already suffered enough.

But the surgery was necessary. Without it, the tumor would continue to grow and further compromise vital sense organs. However, she did not shrink from the necessary surgery, she generated strength for it. She gathered family, entrusted the doctors, prayed, and felt peace. During a long day's surgery, friends and relatives camped out, called, and text-messaged. When the lead surgeon reported C.H. was in recovery, everybody grabbed cell phones. Moved to SICU, C. H.'s nurse brought her a grape Popsicle. She had never liked grape-flavored anything. "Thanks, do you have orange, instead?" she asked brightly, just two hours out of surgery.

The surgeons removed the tumor. C.H. lost the ability to hear out of her right ear. Once home, she began doing exercises to restore some sense of balance. The exercise regimen took perseverance. Trying to balance herself with eyes closed while standing on one leg, she fell over week after week. But she was determined. After several months, she started taking walks around the block. They were short at first, and wobbly. They aren't any longer. Her walking is characteristic of what moves her and who she is.

Six years after her surgery and past sixty, C. H. walks four miles in an hour at least five or six times a week. She loves to travel, dotes on her two grandchildren, and has taken up golf. She stretches daily, exercises, and out walks her husband and adult children on her favorite North Carolina beach. In C.H., what you see is what you get: hopefulness, optimism, and unaffected wonder. She is a believer in all things possible, large and small. She is prayerful and spiritually centered, and a family lover, soul connector, and abiding friend. Today, the only thing different about C.H. since surgery is this: you have to stand or sit on her left if you want her to hear you. Other than that, her laughter is still infectious, and her spirit and zest for life remain as true as in childhood days when she shouted, "Look at me," then fell off the swing. Now, as then, C.H. embraces her life and imagines it well.

THE SOUL LINK

When you are hurting, there is always more to you than a mind needing readjustment or a body part needing to be fixed. When you feel well, there is more to you than merely an attitude adjustment or repaired parts.

In sickness and in health, within you is an abiding, though sometimes neglected, inner life.

It abides in you this side of unconsciousness, but a shade past full comprehension. You know it less by being able to define it than you do by being able to feel it, especially in its impassioned, inspired, arduous, or playful demonstrations. Stirred, it sparks rhythm and rhyme within you. Moved, it provides an empathetic nudge, a deep sigh, a deep peace, and a harmony with the environment. However, when ignored, neglected, or bruised, the soul declares its own unique aching and yearning.

Paradoxically, it is manifest in both the height and depth of your being. It seeks the transcendent, yet foments an undertow, a pull of its murkier currents. It is your inner life—*soul*, as some would say.

Are we using religious talk here? For some of you, we likely are. We realize that using terms like *inner life* and *soul* may connote specific religious meaning to some readers, and broad spiritual meaning to others. The connotations may be positive or negative, depending upon your point of view. Therefore, we want to say what we do not mean by inner life and soul. In using these terms, it is not our intent to promote or critique any particular religious dogma or type of spirituality. With our emphasis upon wholeness, we are clearly not referring to soul or inner life as the dualistic opposite of body. Instead, we are referring to an integral facet of the whole you.

Nevertheless, we appreciate that the word *soul* may carry baggage. Therefore, we will also use the term *inner life*, not as some new age musing on spirituality, but as what we perceive to be a personal, life-encompassing interior reality.

In our vocational practices and daily life experiences, we see that people sense what you sense inside yourself. You know that within you there are more than cells, tissue, visceral organs, and other body parts. Your heart is more than a pump made out of muscle. Your gut is more than a digestive and waste management system. Your mind/brain is more than billions of neurons. You've thought about, intuited, felt, and sensed that *more*, even if you haven't been able to articulate it.

Stirred by a song or moved by a scene, your body chemistry kicks into gear. Waiting in anticipation, your gut may tingle, your mind trip a memory, and your heart pick up the pace, but there is something more going on. Something connects you to the music or the scene. Some tie binds you to the moment. There is movement, harmony, and rhythm between and within.

This is the inner life's crafting, the ties and threads that knit together inspiration, intimation, wonder, mind/brain and body, and the world. It does not use the tool of *understanding*, because what moves you is often beyond understanding. Instead, the inner life uses imagination as its implement—your imagination.

Imagine a favorite spot miles away from where you now sit and read. See its waters, hills, beaches, or forests. Take in its vistas and scents. Recapture a long ago song. Hear the oldie, aria, or big band sound. Listen to the voices of the past. Taste summer comfort food and feel the sun even as the snow falls. This is your imagination at work, creating and re-creating as you wonder and as it wills. Once, it was your childhood escort introducing you to imaginary companions and secret worlds.

However, when symptomatic, you fear its numbing lifelessness or loss. You doubt your ability to imagine much, let alone imagine yourself well. The undertow of your inner life is disquieting. Images and voices you try to recall are hazy and faint. This is disturbing but understandable.

Turn back to Thomas Moore's quote at the beginning of the chapter. From our professional experience, we share his assessment that symptoms often present themselves in areas bereft of imagination.

There is a link between a dulled inner life and your symptoms.

We will explore what it is in **PART 3**, and in **PART 4**, provide a strategy for rekindling your inner life and finding health. For now, hold onto this:

Your inner life abides even when you lose touch with it. The numbness can be thawed, the dullness sharpened. With patience and practice, you can imagine well again.

Are you beginning to see differently?

LINK

Turn to **PART 3**, where you will see that the very systems meant to provide stability and balance can produce symptoms, illness, and disease when they are out of sync and imbalanced. In Chapters 13 and 14, you will learn *how* your symptoms emerge. Then, in Chapters 15 through 18, you will discover *why*.

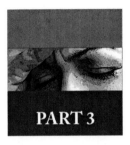

PART 3

The Imbalanced Self

CHAPTER 13

We Are All Symptomatic:
A New Model of Disease

QUESTIONS

What's behind the symptoms? What's behind the hurt?

QUOTES

"The first stage of healing always begins with breakdown. The first stage of healing is characterized by a focus on, and attention to, the external manifestations of distress (symptoms)."

Intentional Healing
ELLIOTT S. DACHER, M.D.

Chest pain, difficulty in breathing, muscle and skeletal pain, dizziness, constipation, abdominal upset, insomnia, fatigue: these symptoms are the bread and butter of the daily practice of medicine. Yet in as many as three-quarters of all cases, doctors can find no disease process to explain their presence, says Dr. Kurt Kroenke.

Reporting in *The New York Times,* June 24, 2001
LOIS B. MORRIS

"Your tests are normal."

DOCTOR TO PATIENT
One of the seventy-five percent of the patients cited above

ABOUT THE QUOTES

At this point, you are already familiar with the research, work, and find-ings of Dr. Kroenke. Given the statistics, can you imagine being a doctor who has to explain to most of his or her patients that their symp-toms have no discernible cause? Can you picture being on the receiving end of such news? Reading this book, you likely can because you've been in this situation. If you got any relief from your doctor's findings, it is prob-ably because the symptoms themselves were only temporary. Dr. Kroenke has reported that in most cases, the symptoms, explainable or not, go away within two weeks of medical treatment, medication, diet care, stress reduc-tion, and rest. What about the cases where the patients don't feel better and/or develop additional unexplainable symptoms? What about you if you are one of the cases? Regardless of the absence of diagnosis, you know the symptoms are real. After all, you're the one suffering from them. The problem is that your doctor seeks objective clinical findings. You can only describe your symptoms as best you can. When the two perspectives are not in sync, you and your doctor struggle with being angry and frustrated. It often comes at considerable cost.

Further complicating matters is the number of unexplained symptoms a patient has at any given time. In an article in *The New York Times*, Dr. Steven Locke, then chief of Behavioral Medicine at Harvard Vanguard Medical Associates, states, "With five symptoms there is a 60 percent likelihood, usually of an underlying depression or anxiety." Thus, as the number of undiagnosed and unexplained symptoms increases, there is even more reason to ask,

What's behind my symptoms?

While initially both patient and physician focus on the symptoms them-selves, they are only the external manifestations of dysfunction and distress.

Mind/brain, body, and inner life are signaling something—some deep need to look behind and look within—in order to discover the truth.

At times, everyone hurts. **PART 3** is about what's happening when this is the case.

CASE PRESENTATION: DOCTOR/AUTHOR

D.A. is a fifty-two-year-old wife, mother, and RN at Mount Carmel West hospital in Columbus, Ohio, where I practiced. D.A.'s chief complaint is abdominal pain and constipation. She has previously been diagnosed with fibromyalgia, interstitial cystitis, and chronic headaches. She has trouble sleeping, and she is considering consultation with a sleep specialist. She admits that she feels unwell and is always tired.

She is five feet, four inches tall and weighs 200 pounds. (I remember her when she first started working at the hospital and weighed about 120 pounds; she's been gaining weight gradually since I met her.) She has developed hypertension, elevated cholesterol, and diabetes. Her gastro-intestinal evaluation was normal, and she received another diagnosis: irritable bowel syndrome. Based upon her response to screening questions for anxiety and depression, she was probably suffering from both. When her attending physician suggested these diagnoses, she responded that if she were depressed, it was because she was sick.

YOU'RE READY NOW

Danish researchers, P. Fink and M. Rosendal write:

There is an immediate need for a common language and theoretical framework of understanding of functional symptoms and disorders across medical specialties, clinically and scientifically. Any names that presuppose a mind-body dualism (such as somatization, medically unexplained) ought to be abolished.

For example, depending upon the country, many people have chronic and recurrent abdominal pain associated with disturbed bowel function. These are the symptoms of irritable bowel syndrome, even though most people with them have not been formally diagnosed. In the United States, the prevalence of irritable bowel syndrome in the community is approximately fifteen percent. Up to four percent of the general population suffer chronic widespread pain, fatigue, and sleep problems, which would result in a diagnosis of fibromyalgia. As you now know, irritable bowel syndrome, fibromyalgia, and other symptom syndromes, such as chronic headache, back pain, fatigue, and interstitial cystitis commonly co-exist. The association of medically unexplained symptoms and symptom syndromes with depression is high, and depression is common. The quality of life is often low. The suffering is often high and disability may result.

Regardless of the reality and severity of medically unexplained symptoms and symptom syndromes, patients recognize when their doctors and other caregivers don't validate their symptoms, don't know how to help them, and don't even want to try. To add insult to injury, doctors may even be disparaging of these diseases.

In a recent survey, doctors in Norway ranked fibromyalgia as the least "prestigious" illness in medicine! (Heart attack was first.)

You know why. Doctor visits can be very time consuming when everybody is out of time. Medical tests fail to show a cause. The double hurt of mind/brain and body described in Chapter 6 is problematic. Doctors are often inclined to attribute the symptoms to stress, depression, and somatization. And to top it all off, the medications they prescribe often fail to help.

We have been preparing you for the truth behind the epidemic of symptoms and disease. You first learned of it in the Introduction. Dr. Manuel Martinez-Lavin is chief of the rheumatology department at the National Institute of Cardiology in Mexico City and professor of rheumatology at the National Autonomous University of Mexico. He says:

"The best way to understand complex systems is with a holistic approach: viewing the system dynamics in its entirety and observing its interactions with the environment. Complexity theory provides a scientific foundation for holism."

Patients, doctors, and care-giving professionals need a comprehensive, integrated, and holistic model of disease. Therefore, we propose that,

Everyone hurts. Life is hard, too fast, complicated, and very stressful; we weren't designed to live this way. The real dis-ease that results is dysfunction and relational imbalance of our complex mind/brains, bodies, and souls expressed as symptoms and symptom syndromes in epidemic proportion. However, by looking behind the symptoms and confronting what we find, we can regain our balance and FIND HEALTH.

Let's break this down.

Everyone hurts.

You may have thought you were in the minority. Now you know the truth. Recall the giant Symptoms Iceberg. Dysfunctional, we are all symptomatic. Symptomatic, we are out of balance.

Life is hard, too fast...

You know it's true from your personal experience. "According to a study just released by scientists at Duke University, life is too hard," writes Ian Frazier in "Researchers Say" in the December 9, 2002 issue of *The New Yorker*. He goes on to say,

Although their findings mainly concern life as experienced by human beings, the study also applies to other animate forms, the scientists claim. Years of tests, experiments, and complex computer simulations provide solid statistical evidence in support of old folk sayings that described life as 'a vale of sorrows,' 'a woeful trial,' 'a kick in the teeth,' 'not worth living,' and so on. Like much common wisdom, these sayings turn out to contain more than a little truth.

You also know that life is too fast. You've been reminded of that by insurance company ads and twenty-four-hour-a-day news. As civilization has advanced, you have taken part in the human *race*. Never in history have people had so much to do so quickly in so little time. In his book, *Faster: The Acceleration of Just About Everything*, James Gleick writes, "Gridlocked and tarmacked are metonyms of our era: to be gridlocked or tarmacked is to be stuck in place, our fastest engines idling all around, as time passes and blood pressures rise." *Hurry sickness* is the term coined in the 1970's by two cardiologists, Meyer Friedman and Ray Rosenman, while researching personality types. Gleick refers to it in his book: "The microwave oven is one of the modern objects that convey the most elemental feeling of power over the passing seconds. If you suffer from hurry sickness...you may find yourself punching eighty-eight seconds instead of ninety because it is faster to tap the same digit twice."

Complicated...

In *Walden*, Henry David Thoreau writes of living in the woods near Walden Pond as a means of "living deliberately." It was his opinion that life in the 1800's was too complicated, so he wanted to simplify things and return to the basics. Can you imagine what he would think about life today? You don't have to imagine what your life is like. You know it's complicated, just as it is for everyone else.

and very stressful.

Are you stressed out a lot of the time?

Most people answer this question with an emphatic "Yes!" It's so important for you to understand and see stress in a new way that you will study it in detail in Chapter 15. For now, accept what you know to be true: life is very stressful for everyone. As stated on the Internet site of the Benson-Henry Institute for Mind Body Medicine in Boston, which is affiliated with the Massachusetts General Hospital and was founded by Herbert Benson, M.D., author of *Timeless Healing*, "Stress can make you sick."

We weren't designed to live this way.

There are two reasons. The first reason is our biological response to living this way. In *The End of Stress as We Know It*, Bruce McEwen says that our bodies and brains have not evolved to respond to the daily—indeed, moment-to-moment—stressors that bombard us. Author of *Why Zebra's Don't Get Ulcers,* Stanford neuroscientist Dr. Robert Sapolsky says, "Stress is anything in the external world that knocks you out of homeostatic balance. Let's say you're a zebra, and a lion has leaped out, ripped your stomach out...this counts as being out of homeostatic balance." Stress for a zebra has a short life span: it's "three minutes of screaming terror," after which the animal either is killed or it escapes to roam the savannah again and feel safe, its stress response turned off. Human beings, on the other hand, have an anticipatory stress response that spins easily out of control, like a car losing traction on an icy slope. "If you think you're about to be knocked out of homeostatic balance and really aren't, and this happens on a regular basis, then you're being anxious . . . paranoid. . . profoundly human," Sapolsky says. The point is that humans, unlike other primates, "can get stressed simply with thought, turning on the same stress response as does the zebra." And when that stress response is turned on chronically, they get sick. Work often involves long hours and can be both exacting and monotonous. Dr. Martinez-Lavin writes, "Modern environment has become inhospitable in different ways. As an example, we have lost the night." The loss of the circadian light-dark cycle is one of many major physical and tangible stressors. It is an example of the tiger in your path. We also suffer with many psychological, intangible, and/or imagined internal stressors-the tiger in your mind, including interpersonal and relational issues, major life events, medical disease, and depression. Keep in mind that your stress response is often activated without any conscious awareness of your feeling stress.

The second reason is our behavioral response to living this way. As Walt Kelly's cartoon character Pogo says, "We have met the enemy and he is us." We must come to understand the enemy within each of us. Not only do we live life this way, our behaviors contribute to the harmful effects of our stress response. WBS asked patients during their initial consultation to describe their self-care plan. Most were perplexed by the question. Some didn't understand the meaning of the question. A few were angered by the question. One patient responded, "What does a self-care plan have to do with my stomach pain?" The consultation didn't go well after that.

Few have a self-care plan. When stressed and you reach for the potato chips instead of taking a walk, you probably are adding to your stress load rather than lightening it. James Levine, M.D. of the Mayo Clinic is the author of *Move a Little, Lose a Lot.* He says, "Our bodies have evolved over millions of years to do one thing: move." He goes on to say, "As human beings, we evolved to stand upright. For thousands of generations, our environment demanded nearly constant physical activity."

The real dis-ease that results is dysfunction and relational imbalance of our complex minds/brains, bodies, and souls expressed as symptoms and symptom syndromes in epidemic proportion.

You pay a price for living this way. One of the central diagnostic insights of ancient wisdom is that most people suffer dysfunction that results in *dis-ease.* When stress responses of the normal state of the mind/brain become overactive and/or mismanaged and therefore harmful, our complex minds/brains, bodies, souls, and their interrelationships lose their homeostasis. Stability gives way to imbalance. The imbalance and dysfunction are expressed symptomatically. Our associated diseases and symptoms reflect our complexity. Each of us has layered unplumbed depths. If before you had only sensed it through your life experience, you now know your remarkable biopsychosocialspiritual complexity.

In the case presentation, D. A. describes what you already know. You are living during an epidemic of associated symptoms, disease, and illness of monumental proportions. Not only are individual patients experiencing greater numbers of unexplained symptoms, there are increasingly more of them. The demand for care exceeds the time that can be given to it, even as the association between symptoms, disease, and illness is becoming more recognizable.

Association is the key to unlocking the symptoms door, but questions abound. What are disease and illness? Are medically unexplained symptoms manifestations of disease or illness? Are depression and anxiety diseases—or are they illnesses? What's behind the association? What's behind the symptoms?

Look carefully here. See differently. We are proposing a new model of disease:

Disease is dysfunction, and symptoms are the expression.

It will serve as a lens through which you will see clearly symptoms, symptom syndromes, and disease.

However, by looking behind the symptoms and confronting what we find…

Recall the profound question that Karl Menninger asks in *The Vital Balance*: "What is behind the symptom?" You met Vanderbilt's Dr.

Clifton Meador earlier in the book. He's going to teach you again now. In a humorous and satiric 1994 essay in *The New England Journal of Medicine*, "The Last Well Person," Dr. Meador writes, "If the behavior of doctors and the public continues unabated, eventually every well person will be labeled sick." Today, through labeling and medicalization, people seek relief from symptoms while ignoring their cause. No wonder they seek treatment rather than ask the right questions. As Nortin M. Hadler, M.D., professor of medicine in the School of Medicine of the University of North Carolina says in *Worried Sick: A Prescription for Health in an Overtreated America*, "The public must come to recognize 'the dangers of medicalization' and 'doctors doing the unnecessary, albeit very well.'... 'There will be no pressure to reform an egregiously self-serving national medical enterprise'."

In the healing arts, we have forgotten where we came from. For all of us, symptoms and health remain confusing. However, by asking the right questions, we can find the right answers for the underlying causes of what ails us. By asking, we raise the ancient inquiry into the integral association of health with the relationships of body, mind, spirit, and the physical and social world around us (the environment). Raising the right questions is only part of our task. Each of us has to deal with what he or she finds behind the symptoms. By doing that hard work,

...we can regain our balance and FIND HEALTH.

As you now know, symptoms themselves can be a door that leads to self-understanding. The ancient Greek aphorism, "Know thyself," was inscribed in the Pronaos (forecourt) of the Temple of Apollo at Delphi. Today, two millennia later, we propose that there should be a sign on the symptoms door that reads, "All are welcome to find health within."

SEE CLEARLY

To open the door, regain balance, and FIND HEALTH, you—we all—need a new way of looking and seeing. You have previously seen that the outbreak of symptoms arises within the context of non-linear complex systems. Complex systems are dynamic. They are not in idle equilibrium. Rather, they are constantly adapting to stressors and changes in both the external and internal environment. You know this from your own experience. Integrating the system are the intricate interrelationships of the parts. Out of these relationships emerges a whole that is much more than the sum of the parts. You are one such system.

Centering and balancing your life are the complex adaptive systems of homeostasis (allostasis).

When you are in dynamic balance, not stress and tension free, but adapting and adjusting well, you are healthy.

The paradox is that the source of your symptoms is also centrally located and involves the same systems, which—when dysfunctional—cause harm.

Look at Figure 13.1 in the **Illustrations** section. When the dynamic balance of homeostatic/allostatic systems is altered, the resulting imbalance contributes to and causes symptoms, illness, and disease.

A NEW MODEL OF DISEASE

We want you to have a new lens through which to see clearly and discover what's behind your symptoms.

Disease is dysfunction, and symptoms are the expression.

The evolvement of non-linear complexity science allows us to view symptoms, illness, and disease in a new way that is reflected in Figure 13.2. Return to the **Illustrations** section and study Figure 13.2.

With this integrative definition of disease, note how all of the boxes converge into one.

The box now includes depression, anxiety, medically unexplained symptoms and symptom syndromes, and all components of metabolic syndrome.

All of these symptoms, syndromes, illnesses, and diseases emerge from a common cause—*dysfunction*—that explains their association and overlap.

In a recent medical journal, Dr. Manuel Martinez-Lavin and colleagues at the National Institute of Cardiology in Mexico City state, "The prevailing scientific model demands that to be a 'real' disease requires structural or anatomic (or at least serological – laboratory alteration)." Thus, medically unexplained symptoms would not reflect "real" disease according to the writers' view of the prevalent model. Commenting further, they note, "If the clinical syndrome (the effect) has no underlying alteration (the cause), then either the syndrome is nonexistent or the illness is psychiatric." From this assessment, the inferred conclusion would have to be that the prevailing scientific model considers irritable bowel syndrome and fibromyalgia either to be not actual diseases or to have a psychological/emotional origin. Dovetailing with all this is something you already know:

Standard medical testing does not show the dysfunction that causes medically unexplained symptoms, because the problem lies in disturbances and imbalance of complex system functions of your mind/brain and body and their relationships.

In the **Introduction**, you read astronomer Carl Sagan's quote: "The absence of evidence is not evidence of absence."

Here's the reality: dysfunction is not detected on medical tests, but the symptoms are real and not imagined.

The absence of evidence of dysfunction is not evidence of absence of very real disease and symptoms. As you will see later in the book, sophisticated brain imaging technologies have begun to reveal the disturbances in function that are not detected on routine medical tests.

Dr. Martinez-Lavin and coworkers conclude:

Disease is dysfunction. Structural damage without dysfunction is not disease. Dysfunction with or without structural damage is disease. Thus, disease can be broadly defined as a bio-psycho-social system alteration that generates suffering and/or decreases longevity.

REVIEW: MIND/BRAIN SYSTEMS AND BODY MAPS

Previously, in studying Fig.10.1 in the **Illustrations** section, you saw the four interrelated mind/brain systems.

While not anatomically correct, Figure 10.1 represents the important overlap and interrelationship of these four mind/brain systems.

You also learned that you have multiple body maps within your mind/brain. Just as a road atlas is filled with maps that represent locations in the world, your mind/brain atlas of maps represents your physical self, inside and out. Having studied your anatomy and physiology – having a new understanding of the role of your mind/brain systems and maps in retaining balance, function, and health – you are ready to discover *how* imbalance, dysfunction, and disease/symptoms emerge.

LINK

Turn to the next chapter to learn further about *body talk* and *how* it is more than feelings.

CHAPTER 14

How YOU Are Symptomatic: BODY TALK

QUESTIONS

Are my symptoms all in my head?
How do I feel them?

QUOTES

"Music is the shorthand of emotion."

Attributed to "Christianity and Patriotism,"
The Kingdom of God and Peace: Essays
LEO TOLSTOY

"Fibromyalgia is a disorder of the central nervous system characterized by the presence of chronic widespread pain."

"Fibromyalgia and Irritable Bowel Syndrome: Is There a Connection?"

MedscapeCME Rheumatology, June 28, 2010.
AFTON L. HASSETT, PsyD and DANIEL J. CLAUW, M.D.

ABOUT THE QUOTES

Music has a way of evoking mood and memories. Some of it, like the big band sound, torch ballads, and swing, recalls a particular time and generation. One of us still can't listen to Frank Sinatra without getting misty-eyed, remembering how his mother reminisced and sang along to his ballads. Classical music transcends time. Jazz has a birthplace and cultural roots. Rock defines an era. Whatever the style, the sound of music triggers feelings in its listeners that can range from feverish to soulful, rollicking to mellow. Music does that to you. You, too, can likely recall times, places, and music associated with your own soulful moods. Those juices run deep inside. They are embodied emotion. When they run amok, both emotion and feelings are part of what's behind your symptoms.

There is nothing imaginary about your symptoms and pain. They are real. Your symptoms are not all in your head.

But your head does matter regarding *how* you feel them, which is the point Dr. Clauw and his colleague are making to fellow caregivers in the Internet-based education offering cited above.

CASE PRESENTATION

C.M. is a thirty-five-year-old construction worker with chest pain. He had a comprehensive evaluation of his heart, which included a normal CT scan of the chest and heart catheterization. Since then, he's visited the emergency room five times. His primary care physician referred him for a gastroenterology consultation. He did not describe heartburn or trouble swallowing, and he had a good appetite. He said that the pain was unpredictable and could be very severe. He admitted to being very distressed during the pain and spent most of the time wondering what was causing it and when it would return. When he has the pain, he said that he often feels dizzy and sweaty and noted that his heart would race. His answers to screening questions for anxiety suggested the presence of an anxiety disorder, but the diagnosis was unacceptable to him. His gastroenterology evaluation, including endoscopy, was normal. His diagnosis was functional chest pain of esophageal origin with possible anxiety.

HOW YOUR SYMPTOMS EMERGE: BODY TALK

In the medical journal article, "How Do You Feel—Now? The Anterior Insula and Human Awareness," Dr. A.D. Craig describes how the anterior insula of the mind/brain is involved in all subjective bodily feelings. You are now familiar with the four interrelated mind/brain systems displayed in Figure 10.1 of the **Illustrations** section.

While all four of your mind/brain systems are involved in how your symptoms emerge, the BODY TALK system is the most important, because it is directly involved in how symptoms are expressed.

In Chapter 10, we gave you a heads up that the anterior insula is a very important component of this system, and that we would refer to it again. Here's why.

Mind/brain and body are integrated in the insula, which is part of the BODY TALK system.

The insula does not function in isolation, because all four of the mind/brain systems are integrated with each other and with the body through the mind/brain–body communication system. Like you, it is a complex adaptive system, capable of adaptation and change. Lately, this little part of the mind/brain has been receiving a great deal of attention. At the beginning of Chapter 10, we quoted *The New York Times* science writer Sandra Blakeslee from her co-authored work *The Body Has a Mind of Its Own*. We encourage you to take a look at it and read an article she published in the February 6, 2007 issue of the *Times* entitled "A Small Part of the Brain, and its Profound Effects." The subject is the insula. In the article, she refers to the brain study contributions made by two neuroscientists we also featured in Chapter 10: Dr. Antonio Damasio and Dr. A.D. (Bud) Craig. She points out that Dr. Damasio, who pioneered the concept of homeostatic feelings and emotions, has developed what is called the "somatic marker hypothesis, the idea that rational thinking cannot be separated from feelings and emotions," and that the insula has, according to Dr. Damasio, "a starring role." By now, the integration and overlap of cognition, feeling, and emotion should sound very familiar.

The article goes on to refer to Dr. Craig's findings regarding the circuitry that integrates the body with the insula. As you've learned in Chapter 10, we refer to this integrated circuitry as the BODY TALK system and, indeed, the insula does "play a starring role." As the article points out, we humans (and to a lesser extent the great apes) have insulas that have evolved to such a state that our system of hearing, interpreting, and expressing, what we called *body words*, functions at a very high level. We hear more from our body parts and organs than do other creatures. And what we hear routes its way to the insula.

Here in the insula, (part of the BODY TALK system), the mind/brain systems interrelate and overlap.

Body words are expressed as *body talk*. Body sensations commingle with feelings, emotions, and thoughts. For example, something tastes bad, and you express disgust. Or you sigh and express pleasure over a caress. Furthermore, the insula even anticipates your bodily needs. With the air-conditioning set at a refreshingly cool temperature, you nevertheless have to go outside into ninety-degree heat. The insula prepares you for what it is going to feel like by beginning to alter your body states and metabolism.

It is, as Sandra Blakeslee's article describes, "a small part of the brain" but one with "profound effects." So then, *how* do symptoms occur?

HOW YOU EMERGE: WARNING! DYSFUNCTION!

Consider studying Figure 10.2 again in the **Illustrations** section. In review, recall that *body words* (homeostatic feelings) originate from all of the body tissues and organs—from all of the parts of the body. *Body words* include: temperature (cool or warm), itch, muscle ache, visceral sensations (chest, belly/gut, bladder, and pelvis), hunger, thirst, salt craving, taste, air hunger, sensual touch, sleepiness, and pain. For your health and survival, it is critical that your mind/brain knows what is going on in all parts of your body at all times. *Body words* (homeostatic feelings) report bodily experience. They are sent first to your spinal cord, and then up to the BODY TALK system of your mind/brain.

When a strong *body word* is triggered, or when dysfunction occurs with one or more of the three BODY TALK system responses, the consequence is *body talk* (homeostatic emotion) that is perceived as one or more symptoms. Thus, for symptoms to emerge the *body word* is strong and/or one or more dysfunctional responses from the BODY TALK system ramp up and become overly responsive (you will find out why in the next three chapters).

Three responses are triggered within the BODY TALK system from which *body words*/homeostatic emotions (read: symptoms) emerge.

1. **Intensity:** Homeostatic feelings are felt more strongly. You hear the *body word* as a loud sound, as if a radio dial were turned all the way up.

2. **Affective and Motivation:** Homeostatic feelings are associated with distress and motivation for relief. You hear the *body word* as a distorted, unpleasant loud sound. You want to turn the radio off.

3. **Autonomic:** Homeostatic feelings are associated with autonomic nervous system reactions. You respond to the *body word* of the unpleasant, loud, distorted sound with activation of the sympathetic nervous system. Dizziness, sweating, rapid heart rate, rapid shallow breathing, and nausea may occur.

Recall the discussion in Chapter 10 regarding the role of the sympathetic nervous system with chronic pain and symptoms. With significant acute and/or chronic stressors, including physical and/or emotional trauma and infection, the complex adaptive system of the autonomic nervous system can become *decomplexified* and inflexible. Inflexible sympathetic hyper-activity can result in *short circuits* in the spinal cord, as proposed by Dr. Martinez-Lavin.

These short circuits are abnormal connections between the spinal cord, which is where the *body words*/homeostatic feelings enter the central nervous system, and the sympathetic nervous system of the autonomic nervous system. They can contribute to the *body talk* of chronic pain.

Allostatic load may result in sympathetic hyperactivity (failing to turn off), which contributes to other *body talk* (medically unexplained symptoms), including insomnia, anxiety, nausea, and abdominal pain. When additional stressors are applied, the sympathetic nervous system of the autonomic nervous system may not be able to respond adaptively (failing to turn on), causing the *body talk* symptom of fatigue.

Thus, chronic symptoms can originate in multiple organ systems.

Let's look at pain as an example of first a *body word* (homeostatic feeling) spoken from some part of your body—say, your head—and hear what you might say once your BODY TALK system has heard the *body word* and generated a painful, symptomatic *body talk* response.

1. **Intensity** (your perception of the severity of the pain)

   This headache is really bad!

2. **Affective and Motivation** (your sense of whether the pain is unpleas-ant and associated with suffering and your incentive for changing your condition)

   I'm really miserable with this headache!

   I have to take some pain medicine!

3. **Autonomic** (your autonomic nervous system)

   I feel hot, sweaty, dizzy, and my heart is racing!

   This *body talk*/homeostatic emotional response from the BODY TALK system interrelates with all of the mind/brain systems (including feeding back upon it).

CENTRAL SENSITIVITY SYNDROMES (CENTRAL PAIN SYNDROMES)

There is an emerging understanding among experts in the pain field that chronic pain, which is otherwise a medically unexplained symptom, is a disease in itself. Its underlying mechanisms may be similar to those of fibromyalgia, regardless of whether pain is widespread, like fibromyalgia, or localized to a specific area of the body (e.g. temporomandibular joint disorder, headache, irritable bowel syndrome, and interstitial cystitis/painful bladder syndrome).

The underlying pain is related to central nervous system dysfunction, which cannot be detected by standard medical tests.

Inspired by advances in the neuroscience of pain, recent research is making strides in ascertaining the "cause" of conditions like fibromyalgia and irritable bowel syndrome. An expansive, more integrative conception of these and other painful symptom syndromes is necessary because each syndrome appears to involve heightened processing of bodily pain and sensory information by the entire central nervous system. Consequently, researchers describe these symptom syndromes as "central sensitivity syndromes" or "central pain syndromes."

We put it this way. By recognizing your symptoms and symptom syndromes as the expression of dysfunction involving the BODY TALK system of the mind/brain, you can see more clearly what is going on.

Let's summarize how you're symptomatic by tuning in to the radio again as a metaphor for your BODY TALK system and see what happens when it is dysfunctional. Refer to Figure 14.1 in the **Illustrations** section. Hear the sound from the radio as your body talk. If the volume is turned high and the tuning is imprecise and imbalanced, then the sound is intense and unclear (**1. Intensity**). You consider the sound as unpleasant and want to turn it down or off and to re-tune the radio (**2. Affective and Motivation**). Your heart rate increases and you feel a little sweaty, even though you may not be aware of these physiologic responses (**3. Autonomic**). The **short circuit** in the radio makes the sound even louder, results in static, and causes the unpleasant sound to persist even when you turn the volume down and adjust the tuning dial.

M.B. Yunus, a rheumatologist at the University of Illinois in Peoria, is the medical researcher who first formulated the term, *central sensitivity syndromes*. He writes,

Such terms as 'medically unexplained symptoms,' 'somatization,' 'somatization disorder,' and 'functional somatic syndromes' in the context of central sensitivity syndromes should be abandoned. Given current scientific knowledge, the concept of disease-illness dualism has no rational basis and impedes proper patient-physician communication, resulting in poor patient care. The concept of central sensitivity syndromes is likely to promote research, education, and proper patient management.

He goes on to conclude that: "CSS seems to be a useful paradigm and an appropriate terminology for fibromyalgia and related conditions. The disease-illness, as well as organic/non-organic dichotomy, should be rejected." Dr. Yunus *sees* the big picture.

COMPLEXITY REVISITED: SYMPTOMS AND BEHAVIORS

The mutually interactive relationship of your symptoms, mind/brain systems, and behaviors reflects a swirling, circular flow of movement. As you now know,

You are a complex adaptive system composed of many complex adaptive systems.

Look at Figure 14.2 in the **Illustrations** section. The interrelationships between the *body talk*/homeostatic emotions (symptoms) and the mind/brain systems go both ways. Symptoms affect your mind/brain systems. Conversely, mind/brain systems affect your symptoms. For example, someone asks you to get up and give your opinion in front of a group. You've never been comfortable doing that. In response, you become symptomatic. You start sweating, gulp for air, and experience dry mouth. All these homeostatic emotional responses and symptoms interact with the mind/brain, triggering more erratic stress responses, anxious thoughts, and emotional distress. These mind/brain responses worsen the symptoms by ramping up the BODY TALK system from which they emerged in the first place. It's a vicious circle. Tongue-tied, you can't think of anything worthwhile to say. Heart racing, you sense that you are rambling and not making any sense. Feeling flushed, you say something, and then sit down.

Speaking of symptoms, in the example above, you said something and then sat down. That's your homeostatic behavior or what we call *body action*.

Your symptoms and mind/brain systems can influence your *body action*/behaviors. Likewise, your *body action*/behaviors can affect your mind/brain systems and symptoms. For better and for worse, *body talk*/homeostatic emotions (read: symptoms) drive *body action*/homeostatic behaviors. Unfortunately, it is often for the worse.

Body action/homeostatic behaviors include what you do and what you don't do, which can have both beneficial and harmful health consequences. They are involved in the *how* of your symptoms.

(As you will see in the next four chapters, your *body actions* are also very much involved with the *why* of your symptoms.)

Action, reaction, inaction, and benign neglect are all forms of *body action/* behavior.

SYMPTOMATIC BEHAVIOR

Do you ever find yourself reaching for and munching on junk food when you get home after a hard and stressful day?

*Body action/*homeostatic behaviors may be seen as symptoms.

On January 29, 2002, the Rockefeller University in New York City presented a public lecture entitled "Stress in the City." The lecture raised the following question:

Did you know that since September 11 [2001]:

→ Drug and alcohol abuse are up around the country (Columbia University);
→ Twenty-five percent of American adults say they have increased, resumed, or started smoking cigarettes, engaged in bad eating habits, or drunk more caffeine or alcohol (American Cancer Society);
→ Snack food sales are up fifteen percent (American Dietetic Association);
→ Surveys show an increase in prescriptions for medications for insomnia, anxiety and depression; and
→ An 'early epidemic of self-medication' is under way (Columbia University)?

Panelists included renowned stress experts, Dr. Bruce S. McEwen, whom we introduced in Chapter 9, and Dr. Joseph LeDoux, whose important contributions regarding emotion we will present in Chapter 16.

You aren't alone in exhibiting symptomatic responsive *body action/*behaviors that may not be in your best interest.

Taking that walk several times a week may help alleviate the extra stressor of paying for those 150 channels but finding nothing on. Conversely, if you lie on the couch rather than going for a walk, you may not be doing yourself and your health any favors.

Are you beginning to appreciate *how* your symptoms emerge?

LINK

Looking at the interaction and interrelationships between homeostatic feelings and emotions, mind/brain systems, and behaviors, you begin to get a feel for *how* your symptoms happen. But *why* do your symptoms emerge? You can answer that *why* question for yourself as you gain insight into STRESS RESPONSE (Chapter 15), EMOTION (Chapter 16), CONSCIOUSNESS (Chapter 17), SOUL/inner life (Chapter 18), and your BEHAVIORS (**PART 4**).

Here's a hint from Chapter 9: remember the tigers.

You've opened the door to self-discovery, and you're inside. Look around and see what it really means to be stressed out.

CHAPTER 15

Why YOU Are Symptomatic:
STRESS RESPONSE

QUESTION

Does stress have something to do with why I'm symptomatic?

QUOTES

"Stress begins in the brain, and apparently only humans can generate stress just by thinking."

The End of Stress as We Know It
DR. BRUCE S. MCEWEN

"We have met the enemy, and he is us."

Pogo
WALT KELLY

"Stress CAN make you sick."

Benson-Henry Institute for Mind Body Medicine, Boston

ABOUT THE QUOTES

One of the great truths of life is that it is indeed very stressful.

"Are you stressed out a lot of the time?"

If you attended one of our lectures or community presentations, you would likely hear us raise that question. When we do, most people raise their hands. You probably would, too, wouldn't you? We know through our education and experience, both personal and professional, that patients and other care receivers intuitively realize that stress has something to do with what's behind their symptoms. Nevertheless, there is continual misunderstanding and miscommunication about stress. People have the misimpression that all stress is bad and that they must become tension-free to be okay. This is not right and impossible. Stressors are a part of life. The issue isn't their elimination, but how you respond to them. Yet stress continues to be misunderstood. Who is responsible? There is no simple answer, but health care professionals and other caregivers share the blame, even though most mean well. A great deal of misinformation is passed down as self-help. We wrote this book for you because we want YOU to assume the responsibility for your health. To do so, you need to understand your symptoms, stress, and health from a different perspective.

Do you recall the quotation from Glinda when she speaks to Dorothy?

"You've always had the power."

It's the same message that ancient healers shared with patients. It's a message we cite with your health in mind. But before you find your power in **PART 4**, you must recognize a power paradox. While your mind/brain and body are geared for health, the way you think and live your life often contributes to your pain. As Kahlil Gibran writes in *The Prophet*,

"Much of your pain is self-chosen."

Yes, you are *under stress*. And yes, stress CAN make you sick, but YOU can choose differently once you understand. Our old friend and classmate, Dr. John Larrimer likes to say,

"It's easy if you know."

But the *knowing* is not easy at all. We know this from personal experience.

CASE PRESENTATIONS

Review our case presentations in Chapter 2. There we shared our personal medical histories with you. Like you, we have been symptomatic. Needing to look behind our symptoms, we both came to understand an important part of the *why* that underlies them. It *is* the stress link.

THE MISSING LINK

Let's look at the stress link. We have proposed a new medical model:

Disease is dysfunction, and symptoms are the expression.

Why is there dysfunction? *Why* does it produce associated symptoms? The following research project identifies a clue.

Researchers have actually documented the impact of stress on the mind/brain. At the University of Pennsylvania School of Medicine, Dr. Jiongjiong Wang and coworkers captured images of brain activity in their subjects with what is known as functional magnetic resonance imaging (fMRI). In research tests, they asked healthy volunteers to execute as quickly as possible several demanding mental assignments. The stress occasioned by the demands of the assignments was caught as a *hot spot* on fMRI. During the assignments, the researchers measured the stress, anxiety, and frustration reactions of those in the study. They also monitored heart rates and alterations in stress hormones. Subjects later commented that they were increasingly "flustered, distracted, rushed, and upset" doing the tasks. During the stress test, they exhibited increased blood flow to the right prefrontal cortex of the brain, an area long associated with anxiety and depression. The increased blood flow continued even after they completed assignments.

These results imply a strong link between stress impact and negative emotional response.

"How the brain reacts under psychological stress is an untouched subject for cognitive neuroscientists, but it is certainly a critical piece of the puzzle in understanding the health effects of stress," says study leader Dr. Wang. "Our findings should help significantly advance our understanding of this process."

Your stress response is one of the four mind/brain systems shown in Figure 10.1 in the **Illustrations** section, which is implicated in what's behind your symptoms.

THE STRESS PARADOX REVISITED

Dr. Bruce McEwen, whom we quoted at the beginning of the chapter, says that the stress response has been around for 500 million years. For both our ancestors and for you today, it has functioned as a dynamic system that helps you cope with and adapt to the stressors of the environment. You studied homeostasis in Chapter 9.

The balance of homeostasis/allostasis (good stress) is essential for your health and survival, but there's a dark side to stress.

A little over a year after 9/11, *The New York Times* published an article entitled "The Heavy Cost of Chronic Stress" by Erica Goode (December 17, 2002). Perhaps struck by the increase of symptoms and unhealthy behaviors that followed 9/11, the author focuses upon Dr. McEwen's concept of stress. She quotes him as follows:

"Humans, on the other hand, are usually subject to stresses of their own making, the chronic, primarily psychological, pressures of modern life. Yet they also suffer consequences when the body's biological mechanisms for handling stress go awry."

The quotation certainly corresponds to Dr. McEwen's comment at the outset of the chapter.

Unlike the animal kingdom, we generate stress "just by thinking."

What's the price for these thoughts?

ALLOSTATIC LOAD (BAD STRESS)

Chapter 13 contains a comparison and contrast between human stress responses and that of a zebra, as described by Dr. Robert Sapolsky in *Why Zebras Don't Get Ulcers*. When chased by a lion, the zebra's stress response kicks into high gear until it escapes or it is caught. Once the stressful situation is over, the zebra's stress response subsides, and it doesn't think about when the next lion will appear. In contrast, humans have the evolutionary advantage of a highly developed brain from which perception, thought, and emotion emerge. Only humans can maintain an ongoing stress response triggered from within.

Unlike zebras, humans can ponder and worry about the next attack. We pay a big price for this because stress begins in the brain, and only humans can become stressed out over life issues that exist only in thought. As you now know, you weren't designed to live this way. Dr. McEwen describes the paradox of the stress response in his 1998 landmark article in the *New England Journal of Medicine*:

The perception of stress is influenced by one's experiences, genetics, and behavior. When the brain perceives an experience as stressful, physiologic and behavioral responses are initiated leading to allostasis and adaptation. Over time, allostatic load can accumulate, and the over-exposure to mediators of neural, endocrine, and immune stress can have adverse affects on various organ systems, leading to disease.

Allostasis can become maladaptive. Intended to maintain your internal stability and balance, it instead produces imbalance. *Why?* Dr. McEwen explains: "During episodes of acute stress, stress hormones provide a protective function by activating the body's defenses, but when these same protective hormones are produced repeatedly, or in excess, because of chronic stress, they create a gradual and steady cascade of physiological changes." From the standpoint of good stress adaptation or dysfunction, Dr. McEwen states, "What is even more important than how we feel about stressful events in our lives is how our bodies react in terms of the stress hormones they produce."

When you are *under stress*, where does the stress go?

UNDER STRESS: RIGHT DOWN TO YOUR CELLS

The accumulation of allostatic load permeates all systems of your body, right down to each individual cell! No wonder you sometimes feel completely "fried."

DIFFERENT TYPES OF ALLOSTATIC LOAD

Finally, Dr. McEwen discusses four types of allostatic load. Let's look at examples of each.

1. Repeated "hits"

This is the unremitting stress that you experience throughout the day and often at night. (Take a moment to identify both the sources and kind of hits you take in a day, i.e., work demands, commuting, interpersonal interaction with difficult people, family obligations, child development issues, cell phone interruptions, twenty-four-hour news, etc.)

2. Lack of adaptation

This is the inability to adjust. Many people are never able to be comfortable with speaking in public. While some people can adjust and adapt if they continue to do it, others are never able to do so. Each time is its own traumatic ordeal. With no learned adaptability to rely on, they avoid it at all costs.

3. Prolonged response due to delayed shutdown

This is failure to hear the *all clear* after the stressing event and responses to it have subsided. One example is rehashing an argument and reactivating the stress response each time. Another is bringing what happened at work home with you and not being able to unwind. A third example is waking up at three A.M., and replaying and second-guessing something you have said or shouldn't have said during the day.

4. Inadequate response

Too little stress response can be as bad as too much. When you have allergies, the immune system goes on red alert in response to usually harmless substances because glucocorticoids and other moderating mediators are not responding as they should. The cytokines and inflammatory response take over and produce allergic reactions.

THE BALANCE OF YOUR STRESS RESPONSE

Stress is indeed a paradox. It's good and bad, necessary and injurious. **PART 2** of the book was all about your balanced self, function, and health. **PART 3**, where you are now, is all about your imbalanced self, dysfunction, and disease/symptoms. Your stress response plays an important role in your internal dynamic balancing systems.

There are three critical mediators of the stress response, the first of which, the chemical messengers, you studied in Chapter 10 as involved in mind/brain-body communication.

1. Chemical messengers

Over time, over-exposure to the chemical messengers involved with the stress response has adverse effects on various organ systems, leading to allostatic load, dysfunction, and disease.

2. Oxidation

You may remember the term *oxidation* from high school chemistry or have heard about the benefits of *antioxidants* in vegetables, fruits, and certain vitamins and supplements. Oxidation is the process of removing electrons from an atom or molecule. Oxygen is very effective in stripping electrons from other atoms and molecules and lends its name to the process. The rusting of iron that turns a solid metal into a flaky, corroded material is oxidation in action. Just as you require good stress, you require oxygen to live, but too much oxygen is toxic. When oxygen and other oxidizing agents strip electrons from organic molecules, which are the large molecules upon which living systems exist, they injure those molecules and render them defective or useless. Unstable intermediates called *free radicals* have an unpaired electron and react with any molecule they meet to achieve stability, stripping electrons from them. Free radicals are constantly produced during normal metabolism. The oxidative stress created by this process adds up. It accumulates along with exposure to other environmental stressors, which include natural and artificial radiation; toxins in air, food, and water; and other sources of oxidation, such as tobacco smoke.

Fortunately, your body has antioxidant defenses, including enzymes and substances derived from the diet (such as vitamins C and E) that donate electrons to unstable free radicals and quench them. Much research is now directed to protective antioxidants that are present in plant foods, including vegetables and fruits, and in culinary herbs and spices. Many other ingested products contain antioxidants, including coffee, tea, cocoa, and chocolate. Whether you should supplement your diet with these antioxidants remains an open question.

3. Inflammation

Your body relies upon oxidative stress, including free radicals, for protection against infection. Infection increases oxidative stress, which signals genes to activate the immune system. Your immune response is responsible for dealing with infectious agents, such as viruses and bacteria. You know what happens when you get an infected cut: an *inflammatory* response with redness, heat, swelling, and pain. These changes are the consequence of the influx of immune cells and blood to the site. It's uncomfortable, but necessary. Inflammation is both positive and negative. It's the cornerstone of your body's defenses against infection and a crucial component of the healing system. However, it can cause and contribute to dysfunction and disease, such as autoimmunity and coronary artery disease. It can turn against the body. This is why inflammation, when healthy, is in careful balance.

INFLAMMATION AND THE EPIDEMIC

The body's ability to store fat when faced with the stress of food scarcity is an example of adaptive allostasis to prevent starvation. However, this genetic advantage has turned into a liability.

Over-nutrition and lifestyles that are sedentary and chronically stressful contribute to the epidemic of obesity and metabolic syndrome. The accumulation of fat in the belly and liver causes chronic low-level inflammation.

In a recent review of fifty-seven research studies, Mathieu and colleagues describe the strong links between fat stored in the belly and liver, inflammation, metabolic syndrome, diabetes, high blood pressure, and heart disease. In **PART 4**, you will discover what you can do to effectively reduce inflammation and the risk of developing metabolic syndrome and its complications.

WBS had a recent conversation with Fredrick J. Pashkow, M.D., a world-renowned academic cardiologist and lead author of *The Women's Heart Book: The Complete Guide to Keeping Your Heart Healthy* (Revised and Updated). He emphasizes that oxidation and inflammation play an important role in several disease states, and he is currently involved in research and development of new antioxidant/anti-inflammatory drugs that show great promise in prevention and treatment of cardiovascular disease, metabolic syndrome, and fatty liver.

DISEASE IS DYSFUNCTION, AND SYMPTOMS ARE THE EXPRESSION

Environmental factors that you have studied may trigger central sensitivity syndromes in some individuals. Studies confirm that patients suffering with medically unexplained symptoms and symptom syndromes often have elevated rates of childhood trauma. Furthermore, the stressor tigers that you studied in Chapter 9 can trigger these symptoms and symptom syndromes. For example, central pain syndromes can be triggered in approximately five to ten percent of individuals who experience peripheral pain syndromes, infections, physical trauma (e.g., automobile accidents), psychological trauma/distress, hormonal alteration, or catastrophic events. Environmental factors have also been implicated in triggering fibromyalgia and related conditions.

So with your new knowledge of the dynamic, ever balancing complexity of your STRESS RESPONSE mind/brain system, let's look at a critical question you've probably asked yourself more than once:

WHY AM I SYMPTOMATIC?

You know the first part of the answer.

The first reason is stress.

There is a clear link between dysfunction causing imbalance (manifested as *body talk*/medically unexplained symptoms) and allostatic load with the bad stress response.

LINK

However, allostatic load does not act alone. Turn to Chapter 16 to discover why dysfunction expressed as symptoms is also related to your emotional mind/brain.

CHAPTER 16

Why YOU Are Symptomatic:
EMOTION

QUESTION

Do my emotions have something to do with why I'm symptomatic?

QUOTES

"The emotions are embodied."

Annals of Internal Medicine 1 May 1997
IAN R. MCWHINNEY, M.D., RONALD M. EPSTEIN, M.D.
and TOM R. FREEMAN, M.D.

Not very long ago, emotion was thought to be the exclusive province of poets... Now, a new science of emotion is discovering pathways in our brains that create powerful emotional memories. Normally these protect us against repeating harmful encounters and guide us to what's good. But science is just now beginning to understand how emotional memories can also become prisons when hijacked by anxiety or trauma.

National Institute of Mental Health

"Emotions define who we are to ourselves as well as to others. They are at the core of many psychiatric disorders, and they can also alter our physical well-being."

JOSEPH LEDOUX, PH.D.
Neuroscientist at New York University and author of *The Emotional Brain*

ABOUT THE QUOTES

In addition to the question regarding stress, we like to ask seminar participants the following questions:

"Who are you?"

"Do you define yourself more by your head or your heart?"

Some people say it's by their head, by how they think. Most say it's by the heart. The heart is the body organ most closely associated with emotions. Expressive or shy, people closely associate who they are with the heart. This has been true for centuries. Historically, many philosophers, writers, artists, and scientists have looked upon the heart as the seat of emotion. For example, Aristotle defined anger both as "a seething heat in the region of the heart" and as a "desire for retaliation." Note that these are complementary characterizations of the same emotion, one a *bodily* description, the other *psychological* (and motivational). You have likely experienced light-hearted moments with friends and gone to a funeral home with a heavy heart. Despite the contrast between light and dark, both describe the same seat of emotion. Joining with familiar expressions like "broken-hearted," "hard-hearted," and "with all my heart," they reflect the broad association of heart and emotion.

Emotion is part of our complexity. Given the widely acknowledged affiliation of the heart and emotion, why do patients and doctors have such a difficult time linking emotions with symptoms and disease? After all, the idea of embodied emotions has held sway for centuries.

The authors of the first quote write, "The notion of the disembodiment of the emotions is quite recent, even in Western medical thought. Classical and neoclassical medical theory recognized a definite medical association between emotions and physical states." Later in the article, they add:

The biopsychosocial model and the patient-centered clinical method require that the clinician attend to the emotions as a routine part of the clinical inquiry. To attend to the emotions only in certain kinds of illness, or only after diagnostic testing is negative, perpetuates the prevailing dualistic distinction between mental and physical illness.

As the quotation concludes, the last sentence deserves emphasis:

"All significant illness is a disturbance at many levels, from the molecular to the personal and social."

Nevertheless, the prevalent trend has been to perpetuate the dualistic distinction between mental and physical illness. Diagnostically and therapeutically, it has been costly.

CASE PRESENTATION: DOCTOR/AUTHOR

J.D. is a thirty-eight-year-old married mother of three children who consulted her physician for chronic nausea. She never vomited and had even gained twenty pounds over the past year. She had no abdominal pain. During an exam, she complained of chronic headaches, fatigue, and poor sleep. She was concerned that she had an ulcer, even though she did not feel better after taking ulcer medication. She wasn't worried about cancer, but she had read on the Internet that she might have gastroparesis, a condition in which the stomach does not empty properly.

She was referred to me for a gastroenterology consultation. On direct questioning about other digestive symptoms, she said that she often had diarrhea and associated lower abdominal cramping pain, especially if she was really nauseated. Her physical examination and laboratory tests were normal, as was an endoscopic examination of her upper digestive tract. She did not have gastroparesis, and there was no gastrointestinal explanation for the nausea.

On further questioning, she realized that she only felt nauseated in the evenings and on weekends. When asked when her symptoms began and what was going on in her life, she acknowledged that her husband was having an affair and was threatening to leave her.

THE PRIMARY EMOTIONS

You already know that you have four main mind/brain complex adaptive systems shown in Figure 10.1 in the **Illustrations** section, which are all interrelated and overlap. You have seen that your STRESS RESPONSE system is in part responsible for *why* you are symptomatic. Until now, you have studied *how* emotions as homeostatic *body talk* (symptoms) emerge from your BODY TALK system and become involved in *how* you are symptomatic. But a different type of emotion emerges from your EMOTION mind/brain system. These are the *primary emotions*, and they are involved with *why* you are symptomatic.

THE COLORS OF EMOTION

What do you feel when you see red, such as a red heart?

Color has a strong impact upon your feelings and emotions. Because this is true, understanding your emotional reaction to color is important in advertising, fashion, product design, graphic design, and architecture. College and professional sports teams invest in and make millions of dollars off the color schemes and design of their jerseys, jackets, and ball caps. Spring fashion shows trip or triumph depending upon reaction to basic black and pastels. Designer paint is all about mood, hue, and feng shui. Correspondingly, your emotions color and enrich your life. They are generated in response to environmental stimuli originating inside and outside your body.

Along with the stress response, your emotions determine *why* you feel what you feel, triggering symptoms and disease. They emerge in response to experience and in relationship with stress and consciousness.

Can you face the truth of your emotions?

THE FACES OF EMOTION

Just as the heart symbol is usually the color red, your primary emotions are often associated with a particular color:

→ **sadness** (feeling blue)
→ **joy** (tickled pink)
→ **anger** (seeing red)
→ **fear** (white with fright)
→ **envy** (green with envy)
→ **surprise** (bright sunny yellow-source TLH's grandson, Austin, four years old).

Because we usually notice the faces of other people first, they tell us more about their emotional state than any other physical attribute. According to Paul Ekman, Ph.D., considered the world's foremost expert on facial expressions and their relationship to emotion, facial expressions are universal across cultures. In *Emotions Revealed, Second Edition: Recognizing Faces and Feelings to Improve Communication and Emotional Life,* he states:

"Our evolution gives us important expressions, which tell others some important information about us."

In these universal signals, we are able to read another's emotions, attitudes, and truthfulness. Facial expressions often give our emotions away, especially behind the wheel, in class, and at the poker table.

BODY LANGUAGE OF EMOTION

As described in the best-selling book *The Definitive Book of Body Language,* Barbara and Allan Pease declare:

"The ability to read a person's attitudes and thoughts by their behavior was the original communication system used by humans before spoken language evolved."

Another overt manifestation of emotion is body language. You can read it in others all the time, but you're not always aware of your own. TLH, for example, grew up in a single-parent home. While he spent only a small percentage of time with his non-custodial parent, their facial expressions and hand gestures are almost identical. Usually, it takes his wife to point this out.

Professionally, we have both been schooled by the body language of patients, clients, and parishioners. Head nodding, eye rolling, shoulder sagging, close talking, tear shedding, hand-beseeching, arms-crossing, and eye-contact-evading gestures speak volumes. What we would have given sometimes for an exam room or sanctuary video camera. The body language captured would have revealed a diagnostic and devotional tale not always in sync with the consultation or "Joyful, Joyful" hymn. More than a few would have been surprised by what their body language gave away.

SOCIAL EMOTIONS

The emotions that emerge from your EMOTION mind/brain system are usually more complex than the somewhat linear expressions of primary emotion, such as fear or anger. The integration of primary emotions into *social* emotions, such as confidence, trust, loyalty, jealousy, and shame, is a multifaceted process. Given its intriguing complexities, interest in the impact of emotion is on the upswing.

A pioneer in the study of social emotions is Northeastern University's Dr. David DeSteno. His new book is due to be published in 2011. He stresses that our complex social emotions are a byproduct of forces of which we may not be consciously aware. On his website, which is available in the **Bibliography**, he writes,

"In *Out of Character* [the book], we attempt to turn the prevailing wisdom upside down by showing that character, nobility, and goodness are all shaped to a high degree by forces outside of our awareness."

Whether or not you agree with Dr. DeSteno, what is important for you to see is how profoundly emotion impacts your decision making and health. The point is that emotions play a role in both *how* and *why* you are healthy or symptomatic.

EMOTIONAL EMBODIMENT

While facial expression and other body language are the external evidence of emotion, most people don't realize they express emotion throughout the internal environment of their bodies. This interior emotion is encoded within you and mediated through the communication systems that you studied in Chapter 10.

This encoded emotion is called primary emotion because you were born with the biological ability to generate it.

Fear and anger have different effects upon your body. In the gastrointestinal tract, fear reduces contractions and secretions (e.g. acid) in the upper digestive tract (stomach and duodenum), leading to nausea, fullness, and loss of appetite. In contrast, fear increases contractions and secretion in the lower digestive tract (colon and rectum), resulting in diarrhea and abdominal pain. This response could be associated with the symptoms of nausea and diarrhea as described by J.D. in the case presentation. Her husband was having an affair and threatening to leave her. Facing the possible breakup of her marriage, she had symptoms throughout her gastrointestinal tract. Fear and disgust produced these symptoms. Like J.D., this gut response to fear has been built in and encoded within you. From an evolutionary standpoint, the response evolved to minimize the exposure of the gut to food and waste material that would otherwise use energy needed by muscles in order to fight or flee. In short, the emotion of fear shifts energy from the gut to the muscles. It comes at a cost, but survival depends upon it.

On the other hand, anger operates differently in the gut. Its effects are just the opposite of fear's effects. Anger increases stomach contractions that can lead to upper abdominal pain. It reduces colon contractions, which results in constipation. With each case, the gut experiences the unique and stereotyped impact of emotion. Fear loosens your bowels. Anger bottles you up. But when emotions come into play, the gut is not the only system implicated.

Your emotional responses are not limited to the gastrointestinal tract. All organs and tissues of the body are involved. This includes the mind/brain, even if and when it doesn't know what is going on.

Now expand your learning curve regarding emotion.

LEARNING TO EMOTE

We quote Dr. Joseph LeDoux at the beginning of the chapter. Here is more of his perspective:

"We come into the world capable of being afraid and capable of being happy, but we must learn which things make us afraid and which make us happy."

Your life experiences, past, present, and future (imagined or anticipated), trigger variable emotional responses that have been programmed in you. You may be conscious of what moves you, or not. Dr. LeDoux says:

Thus, it is possible for emotions to be triggered in us without the cortex knowing exactly what is going on. For many of us, this happens all the time. In some people, this may be especially strong, so their emotions are being triggered in ways that prevent them from having insight into what they are doing.

Sooner, rather than later, you need that insight into what is going on. By way of example, let's take a closer look at the emotion of fear.

IS THAT A SNAKE? THE FEAR EMOTION

The most carefully studied emotion is fear. The EMOTION system of the mind/brain responsible for processing fear includes the amygdala, two almond-shaped networks (systems) located on either side of the brain.

Imagine that you are walking through the woods. Suddenly, you stop. There is a snake in your path only a few feet ahead. Out of fear, your heart races, muscles tense, and all of your senses go on high alert. Then you realize that you have mistaken a stick for a snake. You calm down, step over the stick, and continue walking.

What is happening in your mind/brain–body during your walk in the woods?

Over the last two decades, Dr. LeDoux has conducted pioneering research into the neurobiology of emotion, particularly fear. Recall from Chapter 10 that the senses send information to the thalamus of the brain, which is a sensory relay station, or gateway. (The exception is the sense of smell, which routes information directly to the amygdala.) So any fear stimulus goes to the thalamus, which then transmits the information to two different pathways.

During your frightening experience in the woods, your reaction to emotional stimulus had two phases. First, you saw something that looked like a snake. You stopped, and your fear emotion prepared you for a dangerous situation. Only then did you realize that the snake was actually a stick. You calmed down, stepped over it, and continued walking. Initially, you were startled. Conscious recognition of *the snake* occurred only after your startle response. You saw something that looked like a snake, and this visual emotional stimulus was fired off to the thalamus for processing.

FIRST FEAR RESPONSE: THE LOW ROAD

Dr. LeDoux discovered that the first phase of your response was effected by the thalamus passing a fast but crude transmission directly along the *low road* to the amygdala so you could start to respond to a potentially dangerous object, in this case, a snake. Your body was prepared to act even before you knew what the stimulus really was.

SECOND FEAR RESPONSE: THE HIGH ROAD

The second phase of your response resulted from the thalamus sending information along the *high road* to the sensory cortex, which, on evaluation, created a more detailed and accurate representation of the stimulus. You realized that you had mistaken a root for a snake. The outcome was sent to the amygdala and to the rest of the body. You calmed down. The point here is this: in dangerous situations, the time saved on the low road can mean the difference between survival and death. As Dr. LeDoux says,

"It's better to mistake a stick for a snake than a snake for a stick."

So am I just an instinctive emotional animal like my dog?

BACK TO MY DOG AND ME

Recall from Chapter 10 that while both of you hear *body words*, your dog does not have a BODY TALK system, which interrelates with the other three mind/brain systems. Instead, the *body words* go to control systems in the mind/brain that are considerably simpler. You both experience primary emotions, such as fear, sadness, and joy, which were discussed earlier in this chapter. However, you also have complex social emotions, such as pride, jealousy, guilt, empathy, confidence, and trust.

Both you and your dog are emotional, but you don't feel the same way.

EMOTIONS AND DISEASE

In 1942, Harvard physiologist Dr. Walter B. Cannon raised an important question about emotions in the *American Journal of Public Health*:

"The question which now arises is whether an ominous and persistent state of fear can end the life of a man."

He was suggesting that the physiology of emotion is an important two-way link between mental states and physical disease. Research has confirmed that emotions as well as thoughts, behaviors, and social factors can be translated into disease or even death. Conversely, disease can result in altered emotion, thought, or behavior.

By now, you should not have a negative emotional response when you see the term *psychosomatic*. It's not all in your head, but clearly your head matters. In 1949, in the journal *Psychosomatic Medicine*, neuroscientist Paul MacLean proposed that dysfunctional communication between the limbic system (emotional brain) and neocortex (thinking brain) results in psychosomatic disorders. There was no ability to test this or other mind/brain-based hypotheses until recent scientific developments opened the door to the study of the function of the living mind/brain.

You are now equipped to understand psychosomatic disease.

Ironic, isn't it, how once deeply held beliefs about the integral relationship between mind/brain and body have a way of resurfacing as cutting edge research? On the relationship between emotion and health, we have once more forgotten where we came from. At least, we are starting to put the pieces back together.

Stay aware of those tigers in your life and why they are so important. There's more to come about them in the next chapter.

DISEASE IS DYSFUNCTION, AND SYMPTOMS ARE THE EXPRESSION

So with your new knowledge of the dynamic, ever balancing complexity of your STRESS RESPONSE and EMOTION mind/brain systems, let's again look at the critical question:

WHY AM I SYMPTOMATIC?

You know more of the answer.

The first reason is stress. The second reason is emotion.

There is a clear link between dysfunction causing imbalance (manifested as *body talk*/medically unexplained symptoms) and

→ allostatic load with the bad stress response and
→ primary and social emotions.

LINK

The third reason has to do with the puzzling issues of subjective experience and self-awareness. The subject matter of Chapter 17 is the enigma of consciousness, and it starts for you now.

CHAPTER 17

Why YOU Are Symptomatic: CONSCIOUSNESS

QUESTION

Does consciousness have something to do with why I'm symptomatic?

QUOTES

"I suspect consciousness prevailed in evolution because knowing the feelings caused by emotions was so indispensable for the art of life." (p. 31)

The Feeling of What Happens: Body & Emotion in the Making of Consciousness
ANTONIO DAMASIO, M.D.
David Dornsife Professor of Neuroscience, director, Brain and Creativity Institute University of Southern California, Los Angeles

"There is no coming to consciousness without pain."

Contributions to Analytical Psychology
CARL JUNG, M.D.

ABOUT THE QUOTES

The quotes tie consciousness to the subjective life experience of grasping feelings and emotion, suffering pain, and becoming self-aware. Each quotation appears to take consciousness and its cognitive make-up as a given. Of course you are conscious. How else would you be reading and reflecting upon these words? Yet Dr. Damasio goes on to say, "But I will not mind if you prefer to give my words a twist and just say that consciousness was invented so that we could know life." To label consciousness an *invention* rings strange, when it seems so obvious that we are conscious.

To paraphrase Dr. Damasio, we do *know life*. We think, we feel, we perceive, we plan, we are self-aware, and we remember. All of these attributes have been tied by someone or some school of thought to the concept of consciousness. How we know we know life, how we are aware of ourselves and the subjective processing going on inside us, have been and remain philosophical, theological, psychological, and neuroscientific puzzlements. How does the firing of billions of neurons translate into a conscious self? Those who have put their minds to the issue haven't agreed even on how to frame the question, let alone what the answer looks like.

Freud associated consciousness with cognitive processes like thinking, planning, and perceiving. Standard dictionaries define it as self-awareness. Other thinkers and texts have distinguished consciousness from self-awareness, perception, or thought. While we appreciate the differences of opinion, it is not our intent to immerse you in philosophical and scientific debate. This we know about consciousness. You feel pain and know you are alive. You can daydream, use your imagination, and know what you are doing. You think, endlessly and incessantly. You over-think and second-guess what you did and didn't do, said and didn't say, and you do all of it daily and in your sleep.

Like the rest of us, night and day, you are aware. You are conscious. The physical hurt and emotional pain tell you that. You are symptomatic.

Here's evidence that you are not alone.

CASE PRESENTATION: DOCTOR/AUTHOR

B.W. is a fifty-year-old man referred to me for upper abdominal pain. He was initially sent for an esophagogastroduodenoscopy rather than consultation. During preparation for the procedure, he volunteered to the nurses that his son had recently been killed in an industrial accident. They recalled reading about it in the newspaper. He talked about it repeatedly during sedation. The endoscopic examination was normal. There were no findings to account for his symptoms.

Two weeks later, he returned to the office for formal consultation. He indicated that the pain had been an intermittent problem for over a decade. When asked about what was going on in his life that might be related, he responded, "I've been pissed off for fifteen years." He spoke of several family problems, and revealed that his daughter-in-law did not allow him to see his grandchild. When asked why, he responded, "Do you really want to know?" He quickly added that before his death in the accident, his son had served in Iraq. Two weeks prior to his departure overseas, his wife informed him that she was leaving him. B.W. confronted her about that and she had never forgiven him.

He knew that the abdominal pain was related to his conscious pain and awareness of separation, death, and loss.

A QUESTION OF CONSCIOUSNESS

At the hospital bedside of a comatose family member or friend, a nurse wisely cautions, "Talk to her, not about her. Just because she isn't responding doesn't mean she can't hear you." Those keeping vigil ponder that, tell old stories to the patient, and wonder whether she hears them and remembers.

A high fastball beans the batter. He goes down, sprawled unconscious at home plate. On the football field, a wide receiver takes a shot from the safety just as he makes a leaping catch. In the ring, a vicious right hook KO's the boxer who has no defenses left. For a while, none of them move. Later, each remembers little about the pitch or the hit or the punch. Only those who saw the blows are conscious of what happened on the field and in the ring.

What is consciousness?

We "see" consciousness as one of the four mind/brain systems shown in Figure 10.1.

Merriam-Webster Online defines it as "the quality or state of being aware; especially of something within oneself." Each of the knocked out athletes seemingly belies this definition. Out cold, they are hardly aware. The comatose patient also poses issues regarding a person's state of self-awareness. For that matter, so, too, does losing yourself in a jazz riff or heavy metal haze. In some cases, *Webster's* definition may not always fit the facts.

What constitutes consciousness has been for centuries a matter of theological speculation, scientific inquiry, quack theorizing, and philosophical debate.

Descartes located consciousness in thinking: "I think, therefore I am." Carl Sagan once quipped that we are "star stuff contemplating the stars." Timothy Leary expanded consciousness far beyond thought. John Lennon imagined an idealized world. Some people associate consciousness simply with being awake. Whatever consciousness is—thought, perception, emotion, feeling, behavior, self-awareness—the concept continues to command center stage. The questions surrounding it are now not only the inquisitive domain of philosophy departments and seminaries, but of cutting edge neuroscience labs and psychology research centers whose hypotheses and postulates you can get a snippet of by reading *Time* Magazine's January 29, 2007 special issue on "Mind and Body: the Brain, a User's Guide."

THE TWO PROBLEMS OF CONSCIOUSNESS

Much of the issue focuses on the many-sided question of consciousness and the enigma of self-awareness. According to the lead article written by Steven Pinker, Johnstone professor of psychology at Harvard, two key problems have emerged regarding consciousness, which philosopher David Chalmers has labeled the *Easy Problem* and the *Hard Problem*. The article describes the Easy Problem as a byproduct of Sigmund Freud's insight into the differences between conscious and unconscious thought. You are conscious of some information (daily appointments, faces you greet, even daydreams), yet unconscious of other mind/brain information (how you hold a pen, structure a series of words, have a heart beat). The Easy Problem is about figuring out how to distinguish conscious from unconscious information and identify how the mind/brain processes both.

The Hard Problem is figuring out why, amid the processing and transmitting activity of neurons, you have any personal, subjective experience. How does consciousness (and self-consciousness) emerge from the firing of one hundred billion neurons? Depending upon the scientist, philosopher, or theologian's point of view, this remains a mystery, a philosophical hypothesis, a neuroanatomical construct, or a matter taken on soul intuitions, and thereby on faith.

THE TWO LEVELS OF CONSCIOUSNESS

Whatever your particular perspective, what can generally be said is that consciousness, for all its mystery, operates at two levels: awareness and unconscious (or subconscious). For example, you are reading our book and consciously thinking about its lessons (at least that is our intention). We also intend that you will consciously discuss it with others and adapt your future behavior to regain balance and FIND HEALTH (**PART 4** of the book will be your guide.) You have a mind/brain that also functions underneath what you are consciously aware of thinking, perceiving, emoting, and sensing. This is your subconscious, the submerged mind/brain level, and it is important.

There's a lot going on in your head of which you aren't consciously aware.

Some of it is straightforward body regulation, like the control of your heartbeat. Some of it, like old, repressed memories and emotional pain, is not. Taken together, your conscious cognitive awareness and unconscious submerged undertow have a lot to do with how you feel, especially as they relate to and are influenced by your emotions.

THE "PAIN BODY"

In 2008, Oprah Winfrey and author Eckhart Tolle led a ten-week Internet class on her Internet site. The course content was based upon Tolle's best-selling book *A New Earth*. Millions of people were on-line. In Chapter 5, the "Pain-Body," Tolle begins by saying:

The greater part of most people's thinking is involuntary, automatic, and repetitive. It is no more than a kind of mental static and fulfills no real purpose . . . The voice in the head has a life of its own. Most people are at the mercy of that voice; they are possessed by thought, by the mind…and since the mind is conditioned by the past, you are then forced to reenact the past again and again.

Tolle also comments about how emotion, particularly the old emotional pain you carry around with you, is disruptive. Together, the "voice in the head" and unresolved emotional pain use up energy, prevent your being in the moment, disrupt equilibrium, and threaten to take control over how you see yourself. Like allostatic load, both the incessant mind chatter and emotional baggage become overwhelming. It isn't mind games you are playing, it is your mind gaming you. You are not in sync, but out of sync, not under control, but controlled by your thoughts and emotions.

As Tolle further states,

"Any negative emotion that is not fully faced and seen for what it is in the moment it arises does not completely dissolve."

The negative emotions remain in the landfill of your memories, and they are toxic. In 1974, one of us received a treasured Christmas present from his co-author's mother. It was *The Prophet*, by Kahlil Gibran, which was referenced in Chapter 15. In the essay "On Pain," he opens with a woman saying, "Tell us of pain." The response she receives begins,

"Your pain is the breaking of the shell that encloses your understanding."

Later, the one responding concludes:

It is the bitter potion by which the physician
within you heals your sick self.
Therefore trust the physician, and drink
his remedy in silence and tranquility:
For his hand, though heavy and hard,
is guided by the tender hand of the Unseen,
And the cup he brings, though it burn your lips,
has been fashioned of the clay which the
Potter has moistened with His own sacred tears.

Like stress, pain is a fact of existence. When life is hard, you ache, grieve, and hurt. Eliminating pain and distress is not what it means to regain balance to FIND HEALTH. It isn't possible. The goal is to identify *why* you feel the way you feel and discover ways to respond well to stress and pain, find your balance, and keep it.

NEGATIVE THOUGHTS

Unfortunately, most of us have a complex subsystem within the subconscious dimension of the CONSCIOUSNESS mind/brain system, which includes well-established *self-negating* programs that run automatically in response to life stressors. These stressor/triggers can be *the tiger in your path* or *the tiger in your mind*, which you learned about in Chapter 9. Because of the self-negating programming, thoughts, beliefs, feelings, memories, and physiology may be adversely affected.

There is another *tiger* that makes life even more difficult. Recall that most people constantly feel stressed. But you might be one of those folks who doesn't *feel* anxious or stressed very often. So you wonder how any of this could be related to your symptoms. The reality is that stress may be activated without any conscious awareness of feeling stressed. We call this unconscious stress *the crouching tiger in your mind*. While the original stressor may be temporary and self-limited, the stress response may be ongoing. Understand that this persistence of stress may contribute to your symptoms.

The tiger is lurking, whether you are aware of it or not.

Even though the danger of negative thoughts is always there, you will eventually see clearly what you can do to help yourself as you read **PART 4**.

CONNECTION OF EMOTION
AND CONSCIOUSNESS SYSTEMS

We have previously referred you to the research work of Dr. Joseph LeDoux. Dr. LeDoux has shown that the connections between the EMOTION and CONSCIOUSNESS systems of your mind/brain are *asymmetrical.* The amygdala of the EMOTION system and the cortex of the CONSCIOUSNESS system intercommunicate. However, the amygdala's input to the cortex is much stronger than the communication from the cortex to the amygdala.

Therefore, an emotional reaction like fear can more easily gain control over the cortex and influence cortical processes than can the reasoned, thoughtful reaction of the cortex gain control over the amygdala.

The amygdala's stronger input may be one significant factor in why psychotherapy is such a difficult process. There is at root a fundamental lack of symmetry in processing emotional and cognitive reactions to life experiences.

Increasing the degree of difficulty is the fact that it is possible to generate emotional responses unconsciously.

In these cases, the stimulus is neither known nor appreciated. An example of this is a panic attack, which has no cognitively recognizable cause, at least none that you are aware of. Part of the explanation for the attack may lie with the emotional system of the brain, which has been set up to respond to what you are experiencing without benefit of thoughtful input from the consciousness/cognition system. The amygdala gains control of the cortex as described above.

But you can also generate emotions by conscious thought. Recall Dr. McEwen's quote from chapter 15 regarding stress:

"Stress begins in the brain, and apparently only humans can generate stress just by thinking."

Are you beginning to see the interrelationships between the mind/brain systems?

INTERRELATED MIND/BRAIN SYSTEMS,
FEELING, AND EMOTION

Remember reading about one of the mind/brain structures included in the BODY TALK system called the *insula* (technically called the *insular cortex*)? It is a very important part of the interrelated you. Your memories trigger emotions because memories of your significant life experiences are stored within the part of the mind/brain system that interrelates with the emotions. The significance of this is that when you are symptomatic, your medically unexplained symptoms may be related to experiences that continue to be associated with emotions that were negatively expressed. While you and your doctor may not have explored this area, you should. Here's the reason.

"The right frontal insula is where conscious physical sensation and emotional awareness co-emerge,"

according to Sandra Blakeslee and her son, Matthew, in *The Body Has a Mind of Its Own*, which you learned about in Chapter 10. The right frontal insula (BODY TALK) system lights up when you feel emotions and when you feel physical pain and strong visceral sensations. The authors say:

The right frontal insula is active both when you experience literal physical pain and when you experience the psychic 'pain' of rejection or the social exclusion of being shunned. It lights up when you feel someone is treating you unfairly. Scanning experiments have proven all this, and the results are profound. Welcome to one of the most important regions in the human brain.

We know that by now you see the complexity of consciousness.

WHAT THEN IS CONSCIOUSNESS?

For all the nebulousness and mystery surrounding consciousness, we still find it helpful to view it as the third mind/brain system.

See at the conscious level and give leave for the subconscious to absorb that:

DISEASE IS DYSFUNCTION, AND SYMPTOMS ARE THE EXPRESSION

So with your new knowledge of the dynamic, ever balancing complexity of your STRESS RESPONSE, EMOTION, and CONSCIOUSNESS mind/brain systems, let's revisit the critical question:

WHY AM I SYMPTOMATIC?

You know much of the answer.

The first reason is stress.

The second reason is emotion.
The third reason is consciousness.

There are clear links between dysfunction causing imbalance (manifested as *body talk*/medically unexplained symptoms) and:

→ allostatic load with the bad stress response;
→ primary and social emotions; and
→ consciousness (regardless of its nebulousness and surrounding mystery.)

LINK

Having looked at bad stress, embodied emotions, and consciousness as contributing factors behind your symptoms, move on to explore your inner life. You may be surprised by what you find.

CHAPTER 18

Why YOU *May* Be Symptomatic: SOUL

QUESTION

Why could my inner life affect my being symptomatic?

QUOTES

"A sad soul can kill you quicker, far quicker, than a germ."

Travels with Charley
JOHN STEINBECK

"An inner life is something everybody has, but we lose touch with it."

As quoted in article by G. Jeffrey MacDonald, "Spiritual growth nurtured within," *USA TODAY* January 14, 2008

BILL DIETRICH
Executive Director, Shalem Institute for Spiritual Formation
Bethesda, Maryland

"It sometimes does take a journey to the edge, into territory that is not always comfortable, to discover the spiritual sustenance we so often crave. The dark forest of the inner spirit may be murky in places, but buried in its soil are the seeds of our salvation."

God at the Edge
NILES ELLIOT GOLDSTEIN

ABOUT THE QUOTES

Some people have blind spots when it comes to seeing the tie between soul matters and health. Curiously, they include near-sighted caregivers who skew or otherwise look cock-eyed at the picture of health before them. Take doctors, for example. Some clinical practitioners disembody emotion, soul-searching, and other inner life activity from the physical symptoms of the patient. By doing so, they continue to perpetuate the dualistic distinction between mental (including spiritual) and physical disease. The reasons given are the usual suspects: time constraints, cost controls, and the diagnostic foundations (and limitations) of their training and experience. Regardless of their own soul-searching, they are disinclined to probe the emotional and spiritual depths of their patients. If Steinbeck's quotation has any resonance, it rarely pulsates through their queries and charts. The shadowy stuff going on in a patient's inner life is reserved for X-rays and MRIs, not for an exam room confessional. Matters of soul are for spiritual professionals. They aren't the physicians' turf.

Some of those whose work does include confessionals and spiritual counseling have skewed vision and blind spots, too. One pernicious blind spot has to do with cause and effect. Both of us have listened to care receivers express the belief that their illness or disease was the consequence of God's will and/or their having done something wrong. They read it in scripture and heard it preached that to be God, God must cause everything, even disease. They were traumatized by the certainty of this belief. Can you imagine being the patient whose doctor diagnoses cancer, and whose faith judges God to be the cause? Where would you turn for relief?

You could turn away from religious practice, or you could switch from a blind spot preacher to a cock-eyed optimist, a spiritual advisor who writes and proclaims that blessings, happiness, and even a cure are yours for the asking, believing, and visualizing. These motivational speakers are everywhere today—on cable, radio, and best sellers' lists. In contrast to their fatalistic, judgmental compatriots, they are toothsome, bright-eyed, and encouraging.

We, too, encourage you to be hopeful. There is great truth in the proposition that your underlying mental, spiritual, and emotional attitudes have much to do with how you feel. Being positive has an impact. However, we have seen too much pain and death to offer you only cotton candy cure-alls.

Pain is real, and dealing with it may take you into an inner, soul-searching self you only thought you knew.

Not everyone finds comfort in a smiling preacher or an unforgiving wooden pew. In fact, what is said and taught in some sanctuaries may exacerbate the pain. The judging doesn't have it right; neither does the cock-eyed optimism. Nor does medicine and your doctor when he or she fails to take into account a good chunk of who you are and what's going on with your emotional and spiritual life.

Don't settle for a potion, a pill, or an elixir. Don't settle for doctors who sell your soul-searching and emotional pain short. You are not without resources.

You can get unstuck, even if you feel you've lost touch with the inner life that once moved you. Your symptoms can be a catalyst. They can be the impetus for journeying to the edges of your soul. There you may discover resources you didn't know you had. With encouragement, you can bring them to bear in confronting what ails you and take a major step in finding health.

CASE PRESENTATION: MINISTER/AUTHOR

In conversation, R.W. seems to be trying to touch something long lost. The hint of it emerges in the way he refers to the past and the losses he has endured. He looks around imploringly and grows wistful.

He retired twenty years ago after a thirty-year career in school administration. Public education had been his life's work. Golf and scotch-drinking buddies had been his outlets. Most, he says, are gone now, and he laments that the more time he has for golf, the less he is able to play. He refers to the nineteen surgeries he has had, including numerous spinal fusions, knee replacements, and pain management procedures for the chronic back and joint pain he endures. His clubs sit unused in the garage. As before, he continues to read—always non-fiction, mostly military history and world affairs. Now, however, he says they are all from the large print section of the local library. He hands over a small print book he can no longer make out. "Maybe you can read the small print," he says. He talks about how the yard work he used to enjoy has now been reduced to watering the grass and several potted geraniums. "The hose is hard to manage with my back." He still drinks scotch, but with fewer friends.

What noticeably controls both the conversation and the terms of his life is his physical pain. He bruises easily. His arms and legs are mottled and scabbed. R.W.'s surgeon has recently told him that his back is inoperable. He tries to get comfortable while he sits and says at night he sleeps in his easy chair. On one occasion, he alludes to his dying. He has no funeral plans, no hymns to be sung, or verses to be read. "Just cremate me; I don't care where you dump the ashes." He speaks matter-of-factly about this because he hasn't considered himself a man of spiritual conviction for a long time.

Growing up, R.W. went to a mainstream church. He was confirmed; but he rarely went back. A few years later, R.W. did go to the edge of the South Pacific where, as a Marine, he fought beach by beach, trench by trench, cave by cave. When it ended and he returned, he was by all reports a stoic, hard-edged man honed by war and unspeakable remembrance. "Some piece of him got lost there," his former brother-in-law says. While each of his three wives was and is a churchgoer and one of his sons is a minister, he has rarely set foot in a sanctuary since V-J Day. On spiritual and soulful matters, he has been mostly closed and shut off, until now.

He sits and talks of how cancer and Alzheimer's disease are eating away at his friends. He is the last man standing among his old high school buddies. A long-time teaching and coaching friend cannot remember a face. As they die, the two to four o'clock visiting hours are the time for final good-byes. Amidst the remembering, he notes that a high school class recently held its fiftieth reunion. He shakes his head in disbelief over years passing so quickly. He was their principal. It was a favorite class, but he didn't go because he no longer drives at night. As he tells it, he tears up, and then shrugs as if resigned. In the telling, he is at another edge, in another murky place, but this time, he is home facing his own mortality and that of his friends. Listening carefully to what he says and how he says it, something is different. Something's changed. The man known as a hard-edged, exact-ing warrior with no known spiritual leanings appears to be reaching to touch something inside him. Perhaps it's whatever he left buried at the edge of the South Pacific, a shard of childhood faith exhumed from sand. Long out of touch with soulful sensitivities, he nevertheless gets misty-eyed during recent visiting hours as he openly shares words of love and loss. Later, he lights up with delight at a family gathering when his oldest grandson reaches up to sit on his lap and touch the "edge" of his soul.

INKLINGS OF AN INNER LIFE

You have an inner life. Whether healthy or unwell, you have one, even if you feel you've lost touch. Losing touch with matters of faith or soul or spirit is not surprising when you feel poorly. The inner life is paradoxical. It can play a role in your being symptomatic. It is also central to your healing and finding health. We know this paradox is hard to embrace. We're going to try to help you do just that. In the preceding chapters, we have taken you through the bad stress, embodied emotion, and painful consciousness that underlie your symptoms.

Now we look at a potential fourth factor behind the *why* you are symptomatic. It is your inner life.

Depending on your perspective, some of you may describe it in soulful, spiritual, humanistic, and/or religious terms. Some of you might not. However you characterize it, it's there inside, and it has an influence on the way you feel. Does it surprise you that the workings of your inner life can have a negative impact on your health? Keep in mind the above paradox. As you reflect, note two other points as well.

First, spiritual, soulful, and/or religious people are not immune to becoming symptomatic. No spiritual discipline immunizes you from illness and disease. If you have been taught otherwise, you need to unlearn the precept that a certain belief or practice guarantees good health and blessing. In fact, that sort of teaching can snare you into thinking that because you are symptomatic you must have done something wrong.

Our second point is to say clearly, this is not true. The causes of illness and disease are not attributable to divine retribution.

The issue is not some simplistic, linear, causal connection between the inner life and disease.

The issue is the way in which spiritual and/or religious practice may contribute to and adversely affect symptoms. We have touched on this issue before, especially at the end of Chapter 17. There, we discussed unresolved embodied emotion. Unresolved emotions produce symptoms. One reason you may be stuck is that you've been taught to suppress (and thereby repress) negative feelings. You may have learned this from stifling religious practices and cultural mores, which stressed nay saying, prohibition, and emotional reserve at the expense of simply being human.

The adverse impact of failing to deal with emotional pain is the persisting apprehension of an ever lurking tiger whose presence increases allostatic load (bad stress).

It is wise for you to take the time to consider what spiritual message your inner life has absorbed. If it consists of stifling real feelings, repressing emotions, and/or adhering to legalistic behavioral codes of "ought, and shall not," you can be sure it is affecting your health.

One example serves the point. Anger is an expression of natural primary emotion. It has been construed by some as unnatural and sinful. The basis for believing this is often some fundamental misinterpretation of a sacred text that is then passed down as holy writ. Take the words, "Be angry but yet do not sin; do not let the sun go down on your anger." (Ephesians 4:26). The misread goes something like "Don't get angry because you'll be sinning if you do." The passage really means, "Get your anger out; don't stew, seethe inside and repress it." This is sage advice because what is truly self-destructive is the denial and repression of what is natural. When you deny your own feelings, you are not being honest. That's the real sin here, not the anger.

Take to heart that healthy soul-searching does not involve putting a lid on what you are feeling, but expressing it and working through it. Anger, grief, doubt, and fear are all examples of basic human reactions, which are often quashed by rigid disciplines and dispassionate religious role models. Suppression is counter-productive and unhealthy. The more restrictions imposed, the greater and darker the shadows grow in your inner life. What is repressed does not dissipate. It intensifies, making the soul-searching you must do all the more difficult, but not impossible.

No one is immune from being wounded and hurt. It is part of being human.

To repress what causes pain is not a solution but a further symptom of something deeply amiss. To neglect or ice over the yearnings of your inner life because you doubt and question your faith is no answer either. "A sad soul can kill you," as John Steinbeck says. At minimum, it compounds your inability to deal imaginatively and forthrightly with your suffering and pain. But you don't have to abandon the soul to indifference because of someone else's dogmatic judgment or your own doubt.

Some whom we praise as saints struggled mightily to keep the faith. Mother Teresa, for all her devoted service among the poor, found little evidence of the personal presence of God in the many long years she offered up her care. Martin Luther often cursed God in beer-besotted rage. Saints Augustine and Francis of Assisi polluted their bodies and their faith in early years of debauchery before recovering an abiding soul life within. Grandmas who have been paragons of true belief in their houses of faith have silently cursed God and despaired over the death of a child or grand-child. Both of us have witnessed this in mortuaries and in the ICU. And no cleric, priest, rabbi, minister, doctor, or nurse has ever been without doubt about the loving nature of the creator in the face of what he or she has seen and heard.

But doubt, whatever else you've been taught to believe, is not the opposite of belief.

It is its co-partner. To doubt, to fear, to question, and to lament is to be human. These things do not contradict or corrupt the soul, but reflect its deepest yearning.

Hurting and pain are real.

In the face of it, faith can waver. Souls can sink. And in the bottoms, in C.S. Lewis's shadowy lands, you wander through dark nights of soul-searching and ask the inevitable question, "Why me?" The spiritual ache and yearning magnify the physical suffering and pain. In fact, they are inseparable. Whatever our cultural penchant for holistic health care, we have remained stuck with a body/spirit dualism that splits us into parts as if heart has nothing to do with head, feeling and emotion nothing to do with mind/brain and body. We say unequivocally, that this is false.

The whole is more than the sum of its parts.

Notwithstanding medical practices that disclaim the soul's province, it imprints itself in both your hurting and your healing. Deep down, it is a vital portion of who you are; and even as you are suffering, it awaits your search. There, to again quote Rabbi Goldstein, you may find yourself taking a "journey to the edge." The soul-searching is discomforting. You may already be experiencing that in your own search.

Illness, disease, and pain inevitably trigger hard introspection.

Depending upon inner life resources, the introspection can breed a brooding dispiritedness that further compromises getting well. Or it can recognize opportunity even among the shadows. The opportunity is ironic because it presents itself under circumstances of illness and disease in which you are most acutely aware of feeling helpless, weak, or lost. Yet, out of this may bud the seeds of tenacity, support, strength, and healing greater and deeper than yours alone. In this regard, we share a difficult quote to end the chapter. Initially, the words may seem hard, even harsh. The point they make appears at first blush to be counter-intuitive. But there are seeds of hope sown into what the Reverend Robert Keck writes in *Healing as a Sacred Path*:

Illness may be good – that is, it may serve us well – if it awakens us to what has been frozen within us, alerting us to the life energy that is stuck, or calling attention to a soul-self that has outlived its usefulness. If we are willing to let an illness take us into our depths, we may discover a whole new life.

A hint of what Rev. Keck is driving at rests in the case presentation of R.W., a man functioning for years with a frozen inner life and a soul-self buried in Pacific Island sand, yet not beyond the reach of a child's hand. As you prepare to step forward into **PART 4,** reflect upon your own inner life, your soul-searching in the shadows, and consider that you may be at the edge, the brink of possibility, of dealing with what is behind your symptoms. Then you can regain your balance and FIND HEALTH.

In your inner life,

DISEASE IS DYSFUNCTION, AND SYMPTOMS ARE THE EXPRESSION

So with your new knowledge of the dynamic, ever balancing complexity of your STRESS RESPONSE, EMOTION, and CONSCIOUSNESS mind/brain systems, let's return one last time to the critical question:

WHY AM I SYMPTOMATIC?

You know most of the answer.

The first reason is stress. The second reason is emotion. The third reason is consciousness.

There is a clear link between dysfunction causing imbalance (manifested as *body talk*/medically unexplained symptoms) and:

→ allostatic load with the bad stress response;
→ primary and social emotions; and
→ consciousness (regardless of its nebulousness and surrounding mystery).

If you include soul as a fourth reason, you have likely experienced the paradox of its passion and its ice. What it dispirits, it also can restore, maybe only when you find yourself out on the edge.

LINK

You have done the hard work of relearning and reframing your understanding of the epidemic of symptoms. You see clearly with a new disease model. You understand the *how* and the *why* of your symptoms. Step ahead to **PART 4** and learn how to assume responsibility for regaining your balance so that you can FIND HEALTH.

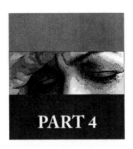

PART 4

Regain Balance

FIND HEALTH

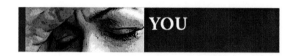YOU

"The important thing is not to stop questioning."
Life Magazine, May 2, 1955
ALBERT EINSTEIN

Remember what our friend Dr. John Larrimer says: "It's easy if you know."
Life isn't easy. So we're going to modify our friend's statement:

"It's easier if you know."

When it comes to your health, you know how important it is to ask the
right questions. Now you know the most important question to ask,

WHAT'S BEHIND MY SYMPTOMS?

You have to look behind them, because your symptoms have meaning.
You know that your symptoms are related to your balance, and your
balance is related to your health. You're ready to explore **PART 4** and
discover various approaches you may use to regain balance and FIND
HEALTH. You know how to see complexity through a clear, big picture
lens rather than the cloudy, one dimensional lens of linear reductionism.
You know that,

Your whole is more than the sum of your parts.

And your becoming whole has much to do with how you handle your behavior. Greg Rutecki, M.D., was the director of medical education, Mount
Carmel Health System, the hospital where WBS practiced. He is currently
professor of medicine at the University of South Alabama Medical School

and an editor of the medical journal *Consultant.* In the July 2008 issue, he writes a commentary entitled "A New Spin on Malthus? Bad Habits and Prosperity Are Killing Us." He references the following quote from D.G. McNeil, Jr. in the June 3, 2008 issue of *The New York Times,* summarizing the World Health Organization's (WHO) recent report on the leading causes of death in the world: "As the world's population ages, gets richer, smokes more, eats more, and drives more, noncommunicable diseases will become bigger killers than infectious ones over the next 20 years." His point is that,

"We run the risk of succumbing to our own success and affluence."

A 2005 study conducted by epidemiologists Mathew Reeves from Michigan State University and Ann P. Rafferty from the Michigan Department of Community Health shows:

"Only three percent—that's three people out of one hundred—lead a healthy lifestyle. This includes not smoking, exercising regularly, eating right, and maintaining a healthy weight."

An important new study published in the August 2009 issue of the *Archives of Internal Medicine* confirms that if people did these four things for themselves, they could reduce their risk of developing diabetes, heart attack, stroke, and cancer by eighty percent! But we know that you're reading this book because you're symptomatic. You hurt just as everyone else does. So here's a right question for you to ask:

OF COURSE I WANT TO REDUCE MY RISK OF DEVELOPING METABOLIC SYNDROME AND CANCER, BUT WHAT ABOUT MY SYMPTOMS?!

Doctors and other caregivers can help you, but the responsibility for your health is yours. Most people don't take care of themselves. Having a self-care plan and leading a healthy lifestyle not only reduce your risk of disability and death from complications of metabolic syndrome, but also relieve medically unexplained symptoms. Because you sense that living in the present is vital to your well-being, you are even more aware of the daily reality of your symptoms. You can allow them to dictate your day or challenge yourself to develop a self-care plan and modify your behavior.

No one magic bullet is going to make you healthy. Medically unexplained symptoms and symptom syndromes require what health care professionals call a multidisciplinary approach.

You can become healthier than ever before and reduce or eliminate your symptoms. Your *body action* behaviors affect your health. With your new knowledge, understanding, and vision, it's possible for you to look behind your symptoms and imagine your health. You can see things clearly and differently. You see *how* you are symptomatic through the BODY TALK processing system. You see *why* you are symptomatic through your stress, emotions, consciousness, soul-searching, and behavior.

You see with the help of a new model of disease:

DISEASE IS DYSFUNCTION, AND SYMPTOMS ARE THE EXPRESSION

Look at the YOU.1 figure found in the **Illustrations**, which summarizes all that you have learned. Take in how much differently you're seeing yourself.

With your new knowledge and vision, you have a better vantage point on your life, your health, and your symptoms. You can regain your balance and FIND HEALTH by exercising your ability to change your health related behaviors and *body actions* to:

→ reduce your stress response;
→ nurture your emotions by lifting your mood and spirits;
→ lessen anxiety;
→ be conscious through imagination, creative thinking, invention, and adaptation;
→ care for and strengthen your inner life; and
→ act in the best interest of your health.

Here's proof that your behavior affects your mind/brain-body relationship and health.

EXERCISE AND THE MIND/BRAIN

Recall that the term *neuroplasticity* refers to changes in the structure, organization, and function of the mind/brain. An article by Eric Nagourney in the March 20, 2007 issue of *The New York Times*, "Exercise: Working Out the Memory as Well as the Muscles," describes a study conducted at the Columbia University Medical Center, which was led by neurologist, Dr. Scott A. Small. The study shows how working out may stimulate the growth of neurons in a part of the brain associated with memory loss. The researchers looked at changes in the brains of volunteers who worked out on exercise equipment to compare the findings with earlier research involving mice. Using an MRI and tread-mills, the scientists were able to see whether blood flow increased to the same part of the brain in humans as it had in mice. It did, suggesting that working out may help produce neurons in a part of the brain that loses them disproportionately as people age. The researchers also found that as the volunteers went through a three-month exercise period, their scores on memory tests went up. "Our study does suggest that it's probably aerobic exercise that's inducing this effect," Dr. Small said.

The March 26, 2007 issue of *Newsweek* includes several articles entitled "Health for Life: Exercise and the Brain." The lead article by Mary Carmichael is titled "Stronger, Faster, Smarter." She reports that the exercising process begins in the muscles, where contractions release a chemical messenger protein called IGF-1 that travels through the bloodstream and into the brain. "There, IGF-1 takes on the role of foreman in the body's neurotransmitter factory. It issues orders to ramp up production of several chemicals, including one called brain-derived neurotrophic factor, or BDNF." It refuels the mind/brain.

Harvard psychiatrist, John J. Ratey, M.D., is the author of *Spark: The Revolutionary New Science of Exercise and the Brain.* He calls the BDNF molecule "Miracle-Gro for the brain." It fuels most of the activities that lead to higher thought. With regular exercise, the body builds up its levels of BDNF, which results in the branching out of brain neurons and the creation of new interconnections among them. Consequently, the neurons communicate with one another in new ways. This process underlies ongoing learning: changes in the synapses between neurons are involved in storing new facts and making them available for future use. BDNF makes this process possible and brains with more of it have a greater capacity for knowledge.

You see that exercise underlies neuroplasticity and improves mind/brain function.

Here's more proof.

POSITIVE BELIEF: THE PLACEBO RESPONSE

A placebo treatment is one that is not expected to have a direct benefit—for example, a starch capsule is given for pain, or surgery is performed where no bodily alterations are made. Placebos are routinely used in scientific studies as comparisons in evaluating the effects of investigational treatments.

Healers have used placebo treatments for thousands of years, and they are often used to treat numerous ailments today.

Like placebo treatment, much of the evidence for the efficacy of natural remedies and herbal products is empirically derived, which means that recommendations and usage are based upon repeated experience and observation. Few natural remedies have been subjected to the rigors of scientific testing, and most probably work through the placebo response.

The placebo response is evidence of the remarkable self-healing capacity that everyone has; and scientific research using functional brain imaging confirms that changes occur in the mind/brain.

From neuroimaging findings, recent research provides evidence that various mind/brain-based therapies, including hypnotherapy, cognitive behavioral therapy, and placebo, all involve engagement of the same mind/brain systems. The placebo response exemplifies the impact that psychological factors may have on moderating the perception of *body talk* symptoms (like pain) as expressed through the BODY TALK system and its interrelationships with all mind/brain systems. Reinforcing this point, a recent study in the October 16, 2009 issue of *Science* by Dr. Falk Eippert and colleagues gives the first direct evidence that placebo treatments lessen pain signaling from the spinal cord. As you know, the spinal cord is the important part of the central nervous system, which receives *body words* before they are transmitted to the BODY TALK system, out of which *body talk*, like chronic pain emerges.

Howard Brody, M.D. is the author of *The Placebo Response: How You Can Release the Body's Inner Pharmacy for Better Health*.

His definition of the placebo response is, "a change in the body (or the body-mind unit) that occurs as the result of the symbolic significance that one attributes to an event or object in the healing environment."

Doesn't this sound familiar? Earlier in the book, we introduced you to Dr. Herbert Benson and his book, *Timeless Healing*. In it, he stresses that self-healing through the power of positive belief is increased by three key factors. The first is the belief and expectancy of the patient when s/he is confident in the positive benefits of the treatment, whether it is a drug, procedure, or other treatment. The second is the belief and expectancy of the caregiver when s/he is confident in the positive benefits of treatment for the patient. The third is the belief and expectancy generated by the relationship between the caregiver and the patient. When both believe in and trust one another, the reciprocal trust increases the possibility of healing. But, there is a dark side to the way you think.

THE FLIP SIDE OF PLACEBO: NOCEBO

Negative thoughts and beliefs have the opposite effect of positive thinking. Just as positive thought and expectancy can generate health and healing, negative beliefs or negative expectancy can have a detrimental effect. Recall Dr. Walter B. Cannon's question from Chapter 16 regarding the mechanism of voodoo death:

"The question which now arises is whether an ominous and persistent state of fear can end the life of a man?"

The answer is YES. The nocebo response can be fatal. But fear not. Take a deep breath. Read on.

RELAXATION TECHNIQUES

Just breathe.

You are now aware of the insightful contributions of Dr. A.D. Craig relative to what we call the BODY TALK system. In a 2010 study published in the scientific journal *Pain*, Dr. Craig and his colleagues summarize recent experimental studies that support previous research regarding the benefits of yogic breathing and mindful Zen meditation for pain and depressed mood. Dr. Craig is not the only one who comprehends.

In *8 Weeks to Optimum Health*, Andrew Weil, M.D., founder of the University of Arizona's Arizona Center for Integrative Medicine, writes,

"Breath is the link between the body and mind and between the conscious and unconscious mind. It is the master key to the control of emotions and to operations of the involuntary (autonomic) nervous system."

Breathing is also a key element in eliciting the "relaxation response" described by Dr. Herbert Benson. The relaxation response is a counterbalancing mechanism to the stress response. It is not only helpful whenever used, but it can also have lasting beneficial effects when practiced regularly. Here's what's involved:

→ Repetition of a word, sound, phrase, prayer, or muscular activity; and
→ Passive disregard of everyday thoughts that inevitably come to mind by your returning to the rhythm of repetition.

Your breathing should be slow and natural while you silently say the focus word, sound, phrase, or prayer to yourself during exhalation.

FROM SYMPTOMS YOU
REGAIN BALANCE AND FIND HEALTH

As you now know,

the translation of *body words* into *body talk* provides the opportunity for true dialogue between the body and mind/brain.

With this dialogue, YOU can discover what's behind your symptoms and take action with your health-related behaviors—your *body actions*—in order to regain balance and FIND HEALTH.

Here's what YOU are going to learn in **PART 4:**

FIND

Find Your Muse, Mentor, and Guide

Imagine Your Own Wellness: Be Open, Unlearn, Rediscover

Nurture Yourself

Dine Well

HEALTH

Hold Your Weight Down and Watch Your Waist

Exercise Regularly

Add Vitamins/Supplements

Learn How Doctors Think and How to Work with Them

Team with All Care-Givers

Help Others Help Themselves

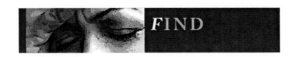

Find YOUR Muse, Mentor, and Guide

From childhood experience, most of us recall that taking initiative is risky. Think back to the days of learning to swim, somersault, dance, or ride a bike. Some of us feared the water or sank like stones in the pool. Some of us never were inclined to gymnastics or smooth enough on the dance floor to do the stroll, let alone the pony, tango, or waltz. No matter how much we wanted to tumble, dive off the high board, or dance, we were stuck being wannabes. Comparing ourselves to those who could, we may have given in to saying, "I can't," and given up taking chances. But those were old tapes about yesterdays.

IT'S UP TO YOU

This initiative is about devising your personal action plan for regaining balance to FIND HEALTH today.

It's about a journey, a process, and taking steps forward and back. You may carry old baggage that weighs on your resolve to risk something of yourself. We carry it, too. On the dance floor, neither of us could be confused for John Travolta or Fred Astaire. Both of us know how difficult it is to break old habits and shake off past failings and missteps. We also know the following to be true. When we did succeed at stepping up to the plate and swinging away, someone was there to inspire us, teach us, and show us how it's done. It may have been a coach, teacher, parent, grandparent, or friend. Someone was there to mentor us and show us the way. From then on, if we really hit our stride, he or she continued to be a role model and provided occasional counsel and advice. But the journey forward was ours to take. It was a matter of stepping up, backtracking, persevering, and finding the muse that would inspire each of us to carry on.

In antiquity, a muse was one of the nine Greek goddesses who governed over and guided the arts. Over time, the term evolved into a broad characterization of whatever inspired someone's artistry, imagination, and creative thinking. Variously described, muses may be mystical, magical, inscrutable, discernible, or plain. They are as diverse as the people who lay claim to them.

When it comes to your personal muse, we are pragmatic.

WHATEVER WORKS, USE IT

That is, whatever inspires your self-discovery, imagination, creativity, will power, and spirit, let that be your muse. It might be music, a remembrance, an image, or a transcendental wisp of intuition. You might be able to put your finger on it and name it, or not. What matters is finding what inspires you, which usually comes more easily during solitude, reflection, the quiet times, and praying hours.

Daily life is full of noise that drives us to distraction. We can just as easily miss the muse. Or lose it.

As elusive by its nature as a muse might be, there are also ways in which people themselves are complicit in losing touch with what inspires them to carry on and journey well. Our personal case presentations contain hints of how this can occur.

During our professional careers, each of us lost track and lost touch. We got stuck in our professional roles and misplaced a larger holistic sense of ourselves. We were determined to make things right. Our self-concepts were tied up in resolving the pain of others. We ignored our own needs and came to believe we were invincible. But the yoke of carrying others' burdens while not caring for ourselves became heavy. When we couldn't resolve or heal, we incurred self-doubt. We doubled the effort. We tried harder to please our professional disciplines. Over time, our bodies rebelled. Each man for himself, too proud or negligent to seek assistance and relief, we plowed on.

We hurt.

We burned out. We misplaced our inspiration. Neither of us could imagine anything well. We were spirit-drained and tired all the time. Becoming symptomatic does that to you. It is also an abettor in the theft of your muse. Muses don't thrive under burned out conditions. If they speak at all, their voices are muted and whispered. You know from our case presentations that each of us experienced significant trauma to our bodies, mindsets, and psyches. In each case, it was a caveat to business as usual, a challenge laid down to self-concept, and a wake-up call.

We had to change.

Under the circumstances, we did what we had been too proud, self-contained, and reluctant to do before. We sought assistance. We sought help in professional caregivers, mentors, and spiritual guides whose expertise, empathy, wisdom, and prayer helped us recover. Sometimes, the fact is that we are our own worst enemies in maintaining balance, finding health, and being well. Both of us certainly were. While it was difficult for us to realize that we were neither immune from pain nor invincible, we were able, with help, to begin to see ourselves differently.

Today, with self-concepts less rutted than before, we remain works in progress. So are you, no matter how stuck you find yourself or how much baggage you carry.

With assistance, you can redirect your vantage point and change the way you think about and see yourself.

No, it's not easy, but we're here to help YOU. Start with two acronyms.

ANTS AND CBT

Recall that there is in each of us a self-defining negativity (Chapter 17) within the unconscious dimension of the CONSCIOUSNESS mind/brain system, which is triggered by the *tiger* stressors (Chapter 9). While the presence of the negativity is a nagging constant, its consequential impact is neither hard-wired nor foreordained. Daniel G. Amen, M.D. is the author of many books on the mind/brain, most recently *Change Your Brain, Change Your Body*.

Dr. Amen calls negative thoughts, *ANTS*, an acronym for *automatic negative thoughts*.

The internal system that produces them is a harsh judge. It is touchy and particularly self-destructive. Think you are stuck with what you are and are not? It will judge that and find you guilty as charged. Think you can't take the risk to look behind your symptoms and find health? It will underscore that because negativism rules. Reinforced by the mental static and incessant over-thinking we have referred to before, your judging self seems to be stuck believing you can't confront emotional pain and its residue, can't stop being symptomatic, and therefore can't change.

But YOU *can* change!

As Dr. Amen emphasizes, these thoughts—these ANTS—*lie*. Do *not* believe them. Here is a cognitive behavioral therapy technique that Byron Katie, Dr. Amen and others use to help you decide whether or not to believe negative thoughts:

1. Is the thought true?
2. Can I absolutely know that it's true?
3. How do I react when I believe that thought?
4. Who would I be without that thought? Or how would I feel if I didn't have the thought?

Once you have answered the questions, turn the original negative thought around to its opposite positive acclamation. For example, "I'll never be able to change" becomes "I will be able to change." Then ask yourself the same questions. You'll find that this exercise results in seeing your negative thoughts differently so that you can take affirmative *body action*.

This is an example of *cognitive behavior therapy* or *CBT*, a very broad classification of psychotherapies, which accents the role of thinking in determining what we do and feel.

Essentially, cognitive behavioral therapy assumes that it is our thoughts about people and events, rather than the people and events themselves, that cause the emotional, physiological, and/or behavioral (*body action*) reactions we experience regarding them. If our emotional and/or behavioral responses are negative, then the point of CBT is to reframe (change) the way we think. The advantage of such therapy is obvious. We can change the way we think about someone or something, even though the other person or experience does not change. Therapy does not overly concern itself with why we think the way we do or with where the thoughts came from. Instead, it seeks to reframe our thinking to change our emotional and behavioral responses for the better.

What does reframing your *thinking* mean for you?

Change occurs by finding other ways to see yourself. You don't try to convince yourself you're not stuck when you know you are. Instead, you admit it and begin to look from different angles at the roadblocks and obstructions you keep bumping up against.

For the two of us, our symptoms were the catalysts to seeing ourselves in a different light.

We couldn't keep doing what we were doing. We had to redefine ourselves in relationship to our work, and in so doing, take a fresh look at how constricted our self-concepts had become. Our worth was tied to our work, and how well or not we made others feel. Much of the rest of our lives—leisure, solitude, kinship, and rest—went begging. Each of us lost track of our muse. Fortunately, as you have learned, it is never too late to change.

Remember that your mind/brain is not hard-wired. Rather, it is adaptable.

You now know that this capacity for the mind/brain to change is called *neuroplasticity*. While it takes work and perseverance to get behind your symptoms and confront what you find there, you have the ability to do just that! Imagine the process like a baby's taking first steps and learning to walk. Imagine yourself as that baby. You crawled before you walked. When you did find your feet, you wobbled and fell down. Often, you were out of balance. Eventually you walked, if only a few steps and likely into the arms of someone who was rooting you on. Reach inward and imagine the scene. Bring it forward and know that you are not alone in this process of regaining balance and finding health. Identify those in your community who can mentor and guide you. Take a baby step in entrusting your story to them.

If you feel you've been there, shared that, and there's no one around who understands or cares, keep this book nearby and visit our Internet site. Read, reflect, and know that we stand by you.

Others are out there, too—spiritual, emotional, and physical caregivers who accept you where you are. Trust this, even with baby step trust, and you can hear again the murmuring of your muse.

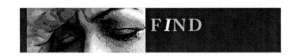

Imagine YOUR Own Wellness: Be Open, Unlearn, Rediscover

His name is Austin and he is TLH's first grandson. Several years ago, Austin fell in love with trains. He watched episodes of *Thomas the Train* on a mini-DVD player that he loaded and unloaded by himself. He also had a wooden train track, complete with tunnels, trestles, and various locomotives, which wandered through the family room. All of the engines had faces and names, like Thomas, Toby, Molly, and Byron. Using his imagination, he directed where they were going and talked to them as friends.

Part of Austin's fascination with trains appeared to have been inspired or at least reinforced by the books he liked to have read to him. One of them, *The Little Engine that Could*, is the story of a tiny female engine that makes a trip up a mountain when older and busier engines would not. When Austin's parents or grandparents repeated the little engine's mantra, "I think I can, I think I can, I think I can," they smiled and remembered the power of childlike imagination.

I THINK I CAN

Both of us can recall when those were motivational words. Thinking that we could do something helped us learn to ride tricycles, hit WIFFLE® balls, and read. As little kids, we believed in the power of imagination. We imagined ourselves as cowboys or firemen. We played with imaginary friends. But the time came when spelling books, rote memorization, and multiplication tables schooled us away from imaginary worlds. Power sources shifted. Imagination waned.

Like the confirmation class in the case study in Chapter 7, we found ourselves saturated with school, socialization, book knowledge, peer pressure, and the necessity of conforming. Play turned into practice and performances in front of parents, neighbors, and strangers who had certain expectations about what they were watching. Just as those middle-schoolers found themselves defining their self-worth by achievements, grades, outcomes, and expectations met, so in our time did we. Like them, we couldn't imagine our well-being apart from our doing well. The intrinsic optimism behind "I think I can" had given way to either self-driven perfectionism or self-verification dependent upon accommodating the expectations of others.

All the while, that judging, self-negating part of the mind/brain vied for attention and control. Fueled by exacting adults, rigid authority figures, and critical put-downs, it thrived. Not only did it dictate the way in which we thought about and saw ourselves, it also helped quash childlike imagination.

You lose the ability to imagine like a child when you become too serious, too conformist, too reserved, too judging, and too adult.

This is a common denominator among those case presentation middle school kids, us, our generation, and you, if you see any piece of yourself in the scenario described here. To grow up, adult judgment must trump childlike imagination, or so in the real world it goes. But judgment without the gift of imagination is myopic.

The issue that arises is this: how do you recover the ability to imagine well?

UNLEARN WHATEVER CLOUDS THE IMAGINATION

Recall the quotes from Chapter 12, particularly the one from Albert Einstein,

"Imagination is more important than knowledge. For while knowledge defines all we currently know and understand, imagination points to all we might yet discover and create."

We advise you to:

Unlearn that you are too adult to imagine. Unlearn the self-negation that you've been taught, told, and bought into that blunts inventiveness and creative thinking.

To unlearn is a curious, seemingly paradoxical suggestion. How do you unlearn what you know? You do it not by whitewashing the past or trying to erase old tapes as if they never existed, but by seeing yourself from different vantage points, by dusting off your imagination to restore focus and gain re-creative clarity about yourself and your health. Depending on personal circumstances, this means you have to take a fresh look at how imagination, creative thinking, and self-image become distorted. Sometimes, this takes you to the doors of those who avow concern for matters involving your soulful self.

In the congregation that TLH belongs to, the children's education director creates and writes the curriculum because she doesn't want children to later have to unlearn what they've been taught. If you have ever been exposed to a linear thinking answer faith that we briefly described in Chapter 8, you probably already have an intuition about what she means. Here is what she is driving at. To imagine well, be well, and flourish, children (and the adults they become) need to know in their bones that they are accepted, acceptable—loved. Most religious faiths profess that their deity or higher power is by nature loving. In Christian circles of faith, this love is known as *grace*. In essence, grace is unconditional love. However, when put into dogma, concrete belief, and practice, grace often becomes propositional. The propositional and conditional nature of what is supposed to be unconditional, accepting, and inclusive becomes evident in the teaching, preaching, and practice of hard core religious concepts.

Some religious groups function like exclusive private clubs. There are all kinds of prerequisites to being accepted. They may be tied to having to worship a certain way, believe particular dogma, or behave correctly to qualify oneself as acceptable, included, and/or saved. Whatever the preconditions are, they are incorporated into the faith teachings that begin in early childhood. Rules to live by are legalistic. The world is black and white. Curiosity, doubt, and ambiguity are discouraged. Rote learning and literal interpretation of sacred texts stifle inquisitiveness and any use of the imagination. The bottom line is, "Don't ask questions; just believe." The net result is the blunting of a child's/later adult's ability to imagine himself or herself as unconditionally loved, regardless of where he or she is in life. How could you when grace is a seldom-heard word?

In contrast, the curriculum director, who doesn't want kids to have to unlearn the legalistic, unimaginative, exclusionary belief described above, senses in her heart and through her creative writing that grace is not propositional, but unconditional. There are no prerequisites. There is room for people wherever they happen to find themselves, regardless of their questions, doubts, curiosities, and out of focus or highly creative imaginations. This is the grace ground she builds upon; and it is worth your time and effort to seek out ground like this if you are spiritually inclined or if at one time you feel you were ungraciously disenfranchised. It is awfully difficult to imagine yourself well if you have been taught that at the deepest, most soulful and spiritual level of your being, you are not well or welcome as you are.

Whatever load you may be carrying, you need to check out, and unload if necessary, any religious baggage that you should not have had to lug around in the first place. Don't buy for another minute the pious sentiment that "God doesn't give you anything you can't handle." To make that statement, to imply that God is behind your symptoms and the cause of your pain, is arrogant and wrong. It belittles and bedevils the human condition—your human condition. If you've heard it said you'll need to unlearn that, too.

To this point, we have described life learning, practices, and beliefs that can undermine, distort, or blunt your ability to use your imagination at all, let alone imagine yourself well. We've also talked about the openness and unlearning it may take to rediscover and regain use of your imagination.

You've already learned that physiologically you are geared for health. You have also learned that you have a flexible, adaptable mind/brain with enough intrinsic tractability not to stay stuck in symptomatic ruts and self-negating patterns of thinking.

The knowledge you've gained is good. But you still wonder if you lack the imagination to see yourself any differently than you do now. Much has happened over the years that may have blunted it.

HOW DO YOU REDISCOVER YOUR IMAGINATION?

Here are our suggestions:

→ **Spend time with children**

Watch and listen. Note how their make-believe extends beyond the constraints of adult conformity and reserve. See how imagination comes into play. Take them to libraries, playgrounds, and children's shows. Talk with them and learn. They are masters of imagination. It may spur your recall that you were once as they are now—full of imaginative possibility.

→ **Uncork your creativity**

If you can't remember the last time you tried something creative, you've bottled yourself up for too long. Try a new recipe. Cook Italian. Taste gelato. Bake. Go to an art gallery. Take time to look and feel. Ask yourself not only what you see in the painting, but also what you sense. Draw a simple sketch or write. Keep a diary, keep a journal, write a letter—even a few sentences on what you observe day to day. Read books and stories rich in description to stoke the senses. Listen to music; learn to play an instrument. Take up a meditative discipline; study the stars. Get physical exercise. Even if it's just a baby step in your mind's eye, take it.

→ **Find meaning**

Patients and parishioners often commented that their work no longer had much meaning for them. Whatever once fueled them to toil long hours had been lost; and the purpose of work reduced to bringing home a paycheck. Many of them had been at their jobs for years. At times, this was our experience, too, especially when we were fatigued and hurting. But just as living has its ruts and dead ends, it also has possibility. The trick is to keep some kind of balance between what is and what is possible. If you sense yourself searching for meaning, stray to the edges of your life. Look around, explore, and travel outside what you know. Go somewhere you've never been. Take a class in a subject you've always been curious about, but haven't pursued. Stretch yourself beyond the cubicle, office, factory, or shop. Invest in others. Volunteer. Get outside your work and routine. Curiously, the meaning you search for may find you as you do.

→ **Feed your soul**

Your soul is the wellspring of your imagination. Imagination is a tool of the soul. By feeding your inner life, you dust off and hone the imagination. Feed it graciously, for you are graced—loved unconditionally and accepted for who you are—wherever you find yourself now.

→ **Return here whenever you need**

PRN is an acronym for the Latin phrase *pro re nata*, which literally means, *for the thing born*. When doctors write PRN on a prescription, they instruct that the medication be taken as needed. So the thing is, we imagine and intend that this book and our Internet site will be an enduring resource for you to use PRN.

Recovering your ability to imagine undergirds the possibility of imagining yourself well. You can sense you are on track when you begin listening to what your body is trying to tell you. Like a private eye, you begin gathering evidence that connects your symptoms to what has been going on in the rest of your life. Motivated by what you find, you are on the road to self-understanding and to discovering the power your mindfulness brings to bear on regaining balance and finding health.

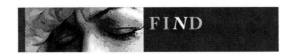

FIND

Nurture YOURSELF

When you are hurting and too tired to get off the couch, you might catch some talk show pundit offering the following self-help advice: "Be kind to yourself and do something that makes you feel good." Reaching for the remote, you sigh and shake your head. If that were all it takes, a warm bath or hot shower would soothe the pain away. While you have nothing against hydrotherapy and soaking in the tub, neither offers more than temporary relief. Your hurting is not something any quick fix can cure. As self-help goes, the advice is too easily presumed. Like bath tub or shower suds, the words simply slip-slide away. With self-care, you have to go beyond skin-deep remedies, root around inside yourself, and wrestle with what you find.

SELF-NURTURING DOESN'T JUST HAPPEN

You can't wish it or New Year's resolve it into being. Nor is it a matter of occasionally being kind to yourself. That's good as far as it goes. It simply doesn't go far enough to insure self-care. Self-nurturing is a substantive by-product of an integrated, holistic way of seeing yourself that does not deny or try to mask your inner critic and pain, but recognizes and confronts them.

However, just as self-care depends upon self-concept, your self-concept is dependent upon what underlies it. Contrary to what you may have been led to believe, a positive self-concept is not self-made. It does not accrue based on performance outcomes, because if this were the case, your self-esteem would be continually dependent on your latest achievement. In effect, your self-worth would rely upon how someone else judged your most recent effort. From experience, you probably already know how tenuous it can be when you look to others to verify yourself. This leaves self-esteem in constant limbo. You find yourself having to please others to please yourself. On that basis, you never quite know where you stand or, for that matter, who you are. As an underpinning for self-esteem, this one's shaky. Fortunately, there is a very different basis on which you may rest assured.

Like imagination, nurturing self-care resonates to mindful, soulful intuitions that you already have the love, acceptance, and validation you thought you needed to earn. You already have it because you are unconditionally loved. This love is the grace we have previously described.

Balanced self-esteem is a characteristic of trusting a grace sufficient to embrace who you are and are not. Nurture is a facet of your balanced self. If grace seems too good to be true, it may be because you have become too accustomed to conditions being imposed on and strings attached to your relationships, interactions, and personal acceptance. In contrast, grace has no preconditions or strings.

Does this mean anything goes? Does unconditional love provide the grounds for egotism and license to do as you please? The answer is "no." Egotism rarely rests on any foundation other than one of its own making. Behavioral license is self-indulgence that has no regard for self-care or others. Here, however, the point of reference lies beyond self-made egotism. It also lays the basis for the well-being of your neighbor because it is solid ground for you both. If it weren't, it would be conditional—good for some and not for others. However, if it's not unconditional, it isn't grace.

This leads us to explore another reason why a first and unconditional love may sound foreign and too good to be true. We begin with the professional observation that many people we have seen have been reluctant to reveal much about the way they really see themselves. They may have talked pain and symptoms, but they also constructed facades. With inner critics chipping away at their self-esteem, they struggled to define themselves.

In consultations, self-assessments, and group exercises, we observed how hard-pressed patients and parishioners were in trying to identify the gifts and positive attributes they saw in themselves. What they didn't like about themselves outweighed what they did. For some, old tapes still played loudly. They recalled being told, "Don't think too much of yourself. Don't get too big for your britches." The admonitions came from those who nurtured them when they were growing up! Having learned not to think too much of themselves, they didn't. Instead, they became used to thinking small.

Curiously (here's a second reason for grace as a foreign concept or too good to be true), there was often little appreciable difference in self-perception for those who described themselves as people of faith. From their comments, the idea of grace had either eluded them or not been mentioned much at all. Despite the clarity of "love your neighbor as yourself," self-love had been compromised. It was as if both the object of their worship and their faith practices were anti-self. Consequently, they had little reference point for nurturing themselves. Whether asked to describe self-care health plans or healthy spiritual disciplines, they often responded with blank stares. They seemed to be missing the nurturing part because they hadn't heard much about loving themselves. They did know how to think too little of themselves and translated that into little nurture and self-care. After all, wouldn't that be displaying too much ego and pride?

The answer is no. On the contrary, there is hubris in self-denigrating piousness, but that's for another book. The point here is that from our interaction with several hundred thousand patients and parishioners, we can tell you that you are not alone if you do not have a nurturing plan or point of reference for it.

So you might be asking yourself:

WHAT CAN I DO ABOUT IT NOW?

Wherever you find yourself, and whether grace is taking root in your soul's imagination or for now seems too good to be true, we are convinced that you can grow into caring for and nurturing yourself by:

→ risking to look behind your symptoms;
→ trying new angles from which to see yourself;
→ sensing that you are greater than the sum of your parts;
→ acknowledging that you can't deal with a part of yourself apart from dealing with your whole sense of self;
→ taking even small steps to discover what grounds your whole being and provides the underpinning for caring for yourself; and
→ beginning to see nurture as a comprehensive and positive mindset of taking care of the needs of your mind, body, emotions, and soul.

Remember, it is not selfish or egotistical to care for and respect yourself. Nor is it a virtue "to not think too much of yourself." The first and unconditional love you seek, you already have. Take this on your journey. Nurture yourself.

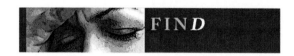

Dine Well

E ating well is both uncomplicated and complicated. We offer you our dining guidelines in the following section.

THE EASY AND UNCOMPLICATED PART

Determine whether you're overweight, how much you should eat each day, measure your waist circumference, and see clearly how weight gain and loss happen.

Determine Whether You're Overweight by Calculating Your Body Mass Index (BMI)

The BMI is a measure of body fat based upon height and weight that applies to both adult men and women. It helps you determine whether you're in a healthy weight range compared to a large sample of people.

You can determine your BMI with an Internet calculator provided by the National Heart Lung and Blood Institute or with the American Heart Association *My Fats Translator*, which will be discussed in the next section under DAILY CALORIC NEEDS. These Internet resources are available in the **Bibliography**.

The BMI is a reliable indicator of total body fat, which is related to the risk of disease and death. The score is valid for both men and women, but it does have some limits. It may overestimate body fat in athletes and others who have a muscular build. For example, one-half of NBA basketball players have an elevated BMI. Furthermore, it may underestimate body fat in older persons and others who have lost muscle mass. Think of BMI as a range, rather than a fixed number like your shoe size. It is best used as a guideline to determine where you are now and provide a goal of what you should weigh to be in a healthy range, if you are not already there. If you are within the under-twenty-five range, try avoiding gaining weight and remain there, even if you have some extra room above your number.

Determine How Much You Should Eat Each Day

You can determine your daily caloric needs by using the *My Fats Calculator* tool available at the American Heart Association Internet site. Entering your age, gender, height, weight, and approximate physical activity level, you learn your average allowable daily caloric intake and body mass index (BMI). You also learn the American Heart Association's recommended range for total fats, and limits for bad fats: saturated fats and *trans* fats. We have more to tell you about dietary fat intake later. Results are based upon your input if you intend to maintain your weight. Write these results down, because you're going to need them later on.

Measure Your Waist Circumference

While you are determining your ideal body weight, BMI, and caloric needs, measure your waist circumference at the level of your navel. You're going to need the information when you learn about metabolic syndrome in the next chapter (Hold Your Weight Down and Watch Your Waist).

See Clearly How Weight Gain and Weight Loss Happen

The formula is simple:

Calories in — Calories out = weight change.

Let's state the obvious:

Calories in is what you eat.

Count everything you eat or drink. The types of calories you eat do not matter regarding weight. Fat calories, carbohydrate calories, and protein calories are all calories. Carbohydrates and proteins are turned into glucose, and fat is burned directly. Some of the glucose goes directly into your bloodstream and is burned for energy, some is stored as glycogen in your muscles and liver, and the rest is converted to fat and stored in fat cells to be burned when your body doesn't have enough food or glycogen.

Of course, you should understand that on a gram for gram basis, there are more than twice as many calories in fat than in carbohydrates and protein, so it's easier to eat too many fat calories. Carbohydrates and protein each have four calories per gram, while fat has nine calories per gram.

Calories out is what you burn.

You are constantly burning calories, even at rest or while sleeping. For example, a 150-pound man burns one calorie per minute while asleep. You can increase your calories out with exercise, which you will be learning more about later in **PART 4**.

You see how to lose weight: take in fewer calories than you burn.

The balance of eating and physical activity determines weight gain and loss, regardless of whether you eat fat, carbohydrates, or protein. It is the number, not the source, of the calories that you consume that determines what happens to your weight. You are going to learn how to enjoy eating a healthy diet that includes antioxidants and is anti-inflammatory so that you can develop your own dietary plan and be healthy.

THE HARD AND COMPLICATED PART: THERE'S WIDESPREAD CONFUSION ABOUT WHAT TO EAT!

Mark N. Feinglos, M.D. and Susan E. Totten, R.D. of Duke University Medical Center write, "We know that as a population, we eat too much for our level of activity, and we are growing fatter as a result." In association with this increasing weight, there is an epidemic of metabolic syndrome. They add,

"… we have to assume that calories trump everything else, and that our number one goal … should be to reduce the intake of high-energy, low-benefit foods, particularly in young members of the most vulnerable populations."

The quotations above set the broad parameter of the problem, but not the complexity. We have found someone who truly understands the complexity of eating. He is Michael Pollan, a contributing writer to *The New York Times Magazine* and a Knight Professor of Journalism at UC Berkeley. As Mr. Pollan says,

"There is widespread confusion about what to eat."

He's right. In his book, *In Defense of Food: An Eater's Manifesto*, Pollan writes that most of what we are consuming today isn't food (it's processed), and how we are eating it—on the run and increasingly alone—isn't really eating. We're consuming "edible food-like substances" that are no longer the products of nature but of food science. He adds,

Many of them come packaged with health claims that should be our first clue they are anything but healthy. In the so-called Western diet, food has been replaced by nutrients and common sense by confusion. Consequently, we have an American paradox: The more we worry about nutrition, the less healthy we seem to become.

Furthermore, he understands and uncovers the complexity and imperfect world from which the unhealthy Western diet has emerged. This environment includes the complex interrelationship of the food industry, marketers, nutritional science, the government, and journalism. Despite the complexity, Pollan answers the question of what to eat with seven simple but liberating words:

"Eat food. Not too much. Mostly plants."

With this, he challenges the prevailing emphasis upon a nutrient-by-nutrient approach called nutritionism and recommends an alternative way of eating that is informed by the traditions and ecology of real, well-grown, unprocessed food. Our personal health, he argues, cannot be divorced from the health of the food chains of which we are part.

Here we cut through the confusion to the common sense, as much as is possible.

EAT MINDFULLY

Dining should be easy, slow, and uncomplicated. For many reasons, eating a healthy diet is important. A healthy diet is rich in antioxidants and anti-inflammatory, so it reduces the allostatic load of the bad stress response. Two excellent Internet resources for learning about eating mindfully are available in the **Bibliography**. The Center for Mindful Eating (TCME) says:

"Our relationship to food is a central one that reflects our attitudes toward our environment and ourselves. As a practice, Mindful Eating can bring us awareness of our own actions, thoughts, feelings, and motivations, and insight into the roots of health and contentment."

The Duke Integrative Medicine Internet site (referenced in Chapter 7 and in the **Bibliography**) advocates mindful eating, which has its roots in Buddhism. Currently, it is being studied by several medical centers and the National Institutes of Health as a method to lose weight, keep it off, and combat eating disorders. "Most people don't think about what they're eating; they're focusing on the next bite," says Sasha Loring, a psychotherapist at Duke Integrative Medicine, as quoted in the May 13, 2008 issue of *The Wall Street Journal* in Melinda Beck's "Health Journal: Putting an End to Mindless Munching." A key is to recognize the host of negative emotions many people bring to the table, like the guilt about blowing a diet or the childhood fears of deprivation or wasting food. Using food as a reward interferes with eating mindfully because if you're eating to satisfy emotional hunger, it's hard to ever feel full. Sasha Loring says, "Ask yourself what do you really need and what else can you do to fulfill it?"

How to Practice Mindful Eating

→ Assess how hungry you are on a scale of 1 (ravenous) to 7 (stuffed).
→ Eat slowly; savor your food.
→ Put your fork down and breathe between bites.
→ Ask yourself how much you really need (for example, a hunger for something sweet or sour or salty can often be satisfied with a small morsel).
→ Check back on your hunger level.
→ Stop when you start to feel full (ideally about 5 ½ on the 7-point scale).

DEVELOP YOUR OWN DINING PLAN USING OUR DIETARY GUIDELINES

In a recent editorial, "Diet and cardiovascular disease prevention: the need for a paradigm shift," Dr. F.B. Hu says that emphasis upon low-fat diets during the past fifty years has resulted in a proportional increase in refined carbohydrate intake, contributing to insulin resistance, the metabolic syndrome, and diabetes. Refined carbohydrates lead to more rapid increases and decreases in blood sugar levels, and this high glycemic load (GL) produces more insulin resistance. Furthermore, the inflammation associated with the bad stress response and the metabolic syndrome is worsened by the Western diet. There is strong scientific evidence that diets rich in omega-3 fatty acids and other unsaturated fats, the natural antioxidants in fruits and vegetables, and fiber in nuts and whole grains provide specific benefit for patients with the metabolic syndrome. This type of diet is known as the Mediterranean diet, which is based upon a broad nutrient profile of Mediterranean cultures.

Bookstore shelves are filled with diet books, and we include several recommendations of resources for healthy eating at the end of this chapter, which are included in the **Bibliography.**

Here are our dietary guidelines, so that you can develop your own strategic plan for enjoying a healthy diet that is full of antioxidants and is anti-inflammatory.

(Recall learning in Chapter 15 that oxidation and inflammation, along with certain chemical messengers are the three critical mediators of the stress response.)

Let's look at the components of our dietary strategy.

See Through the Complexity

Remain conscious of the complexity. See through the lens of complex systems rather than linear reductionism. Understand that a healthy diet is one facet of the bigger picture regarding self-care. While in part, "you are what you eat," diet alone cannot be the single straight-line to health. Furthermore, there is no dietary magic bullet. No single dietary factor or component, either included or excluded, will make you whole. Remember Pollan's advice?

"Eat food. Not too much. Mostly plants."

This is his first line in "Unhappy Meals" in *The New York Times Magazine* (January 28, 2007) and in his book *In Defense of Food: An Eater's Manifesto*. Here's what he means.

Eat Mostly Unprocessed Food

When Pollan says, "Eat food," he means mainly unprocessed food. He advises avoiding food products that contain unfamiliar ingredients, number more than five, or that contain high-fructose corn syrup. While none of these ingredient aspects are necessarily harmful in and of themselves, all reliably indicate that foods have been highly processed.

In general, the periphery of the supermarket has the fresh food—produce, dairy, meat, and fish—while the center aisles contain processed food products. The farmer's market is even better, because you aren't likely to find elaborately processed food there. Fast food is processed food. Enough said.

Eat Smaller Portions of Healthy Food

Eating *not so much* is good for you. Pollan says that for a century the American food system has devoted its energies and policies to reducing price and increasing quantity rather than improving quality. Better food, measured by taste or nutritional quality (which often correspond), and well grown in good soils (whether certified organic or not), costs more because it has been grown or raised less intensively and with more care. Pollan writes that calorie restriction has repeatedly been shown to slow aging in animals, and many researchers (including Walter Willett, the Harvard epidemiologist), believe it offers the single strongest link between diet and cancer prevention.

Most of us need to lose weight and then maintain a healthy weight.

We recommend you consider using one or two tricks to reduce your calories. Do one or both of the following about twenty minutes before you eat.

→ Eat about 50 to 100 calories (75 on average) of *good fat*.

For example, a small handful of nuts (e.g., six walnuts, twelve almonds, or twenty peanuts) or a small piece of whole grain bread dipped in canola or olive oil will work well. Eating fat stimulates the production of cholecystokinin (CCK), which is a chemical messenger—remember what you learned in **PART 2** about them—produced by your gut in response to food. It takes about twenty minutes for CCK to tell your brain you've had enough to eat and to keep you full by slowing down the emptying of your stomach. Then when you sit down to eat, you will be more likely to eat for pleasure than for hunger. You'll be more likely to eat less, particularly if you employ mindful eating.

→ Consider including some fiber with the first trick, because fiber is filling. In addition to the nuts or whole-grain bread, we recommend a psyllium-containing fiber supplement, as we will discuss in the section on fiber.

Eat Mainly Plants

Remember what Pollan says, "Eat mostly plants. Especially leaves." The benefit of a plant-based diet is the only point of universal consensus among nutrition experts. The plant-based diet is clearly good for you, even though it's not clear why. Is it the antioxidants; fiber; and/or omega-3s? No one is certain. But by eating a plant-based diet, you consume far fewer calories, since plant foods (except seeds) are typically less energy dense than other things you might eat. Vegetarians are healthier than carnivores, but near vegetarians (flexitarians) are as healthy as vegetarians.

Eat Complex Carbohydrates and Fewer Simple Carbohydrates

Don't simply *cut the carbs*. Shift from simple refined carbohydrates (such as sugar, white flour, white rice, and high-fructose corn syrup) and rapidly digested starches (such as potatoes and white rice) to more unrefined complex carbohydrates, such as whole grains (e.g., whole-wheat bread and brown rice), legumes, soy products, vegetables, and fruit. They provide longer-lasting energy and lower your risk of metabolic syndrome, diabetes, and heart disease.

With whole grains, look for the word *whole* in the ingredient statement and be sure that the whole grain appears relatively high, preferably first, on the list. A product claiming that it is made with whole grains may actually be made mostly with refined grains.

Eat Five to Nine Servings of Vegetables and Fruits Each Day

Most vegetables and fruits are unprocessed low calorie foods that you can eat in large quantities. They are the most effective foods for health and disease prevention. Don't count potatoes and French fries. There is a correlation between the color pigments in vegetables and fruits and the level of healthful compounds and constituents they contain. When you go to the grocery store, shop for vegetables and fruits that have a variety of color, like green, orange, purple, red, white, and yellow. For more information, visit the Internet site for the Centers for Disease Control and Prevention: Eat a Variety of Fruits and Vegetables Every Day, which is included in the **Bibliography**.

Understand Fats, and Then Plan Their Intake

Things get quite a bit more complicated when it comes to fat. The reasons are, well, complicated. Read *In Defense of Food*, if you want the gory details. One important reason is known as *the lipid hypothesis*. This hypothesis proposes that dietary fat is responsible for much chronic disease. Based upon this hypothesis, there has been a thirty-year effort to reform the food supply and our eating habits. Without going into detail, the relationship of food with health is much more complicated than an isolated focus upon fat.

However, our health is clearly related to the Western diet, which is complicated.

Metabolic syndrome, heart disease, and many types of cancer can be directly traced to the industrialization of our food and the Western diet. Pollan attributes this to the rise of highly processed foods and refined grains, the use of chemicals to raise plants and animals in enormous monocultures, the plethora of cheap calories of sugar and fat made by modern agriculture, and the narrowing of the biological diversity of our diet to a few staple crops (wheat, corn, and soy). As a result, the Western diet that most of us eat includes lots of processed food, meat, added sugar, and fat. Conversely, the Western diet that most of us eat does not include vegetables, fruits, and whole grain.

The whole of your diet is much more than the sum of its parts (food and nutrients). See your diet through the big picture lens of complexity rather than through a narrow, nutrient-by-nutrient focus. This is especially true with fats.

You learned about the cells of your body in Chapter 10. You need fat to provide fuel for your cells and the raw materials for building the cell membranes. Approximately sixty percent of the brain is fat.

There are four major fats in the foods that you eat. Saturated fats, trans fats, monounsaturated fats, and polyunsaturated fats. Two are bad. Two are good.

Bad Fats

There are two bad fats: saturated fats and *trans* fats. The bad fats tend to be more solid at room temperature (like a stick of butter). The good fats, monounsaturated and polyunsaturated fat, tend to be more liquid (like vegetable oil and olive oil).

Saturated Fats (LIMIT)

Saturated fats raise LDH (bad) cholesterol, and most people should limit intake. The main sources of saturated fat are animal products, including fatty meat, un-skinned poultry, dairy products (except non-fat dairy), many baked goods, fried foods, and coconut oil (which is the only significant plant source of saturated fat). Look on the product label to determine the amount of saturated fat in grams.

Trans Fat, Also Called Hydrogenated or Partially Hydrogenated Fat (AVOID)

Avoid *trans* fats, because they are even worse for you than saturated fat, not only raising LDH (bad) cholesterol but also lowering HDL (good) cholesterol. *Trans* fats raise inflammatory factors in the blood and are strongly linked with heart disease and the risk of developing metabolic syndrome. *Trans* fat is a vegetable oil that has been turned into a solid fat (e.g., shortening or margarine) by heating it with hydrogen. This process is called hydrogenation.

There is no safe amount of trans fat in the diet.

Don't eat any products that list partially hydrogenated or hydrogenated oil as an ingredient, regardless of the oil. These fats are found in fried and processed foods, such as cakes, cookies, and snack foods. Look at the label. Look for a "0" in the Trans Fat box. Be aware that the label may say "zero grams trans fat," even if partially hydrogenated oils are used, as long as the food contains less than half a gram per serving. Even though this is better than a larger amount, the best choice is no trans fat at all (eating several servings could add up to several grams of trans fat).

Good Fats

There are two good fats: monounsaturated fats and polyunsaturated fats. By substituting good fats for bad, LDL (bad) cholesterol levels can be lowered and the risk for developing heart and vascular disease can be reduced.

Monounsaturated Fat

Monounsaturated fats include olive oil, canola oil, peanut oil, cashews, almonds, peanuts, and most other nuts, peanut butter, and avocados. Monounsaturated vegetable oils are preferable to polyunsaturated vegetable oils.

Polyunsaturated Fats

Polyunsaturated fats include vegetable oils (corn, soybean, safflower, and cottonseed), legumes (including soybeans and soy products), fatty fish (such as salmon and tuna), olives and olive oil, canola oil, nuts, and poultry fat. It's advisable to limit use of polyunsaturated vegetable oils.

Polyunsaturated Fatty Acids (PUFAS): The Essential Fatty Acids

The PUFAs are polyunsaturated fats that cannot be made by the body and must be obtained from the diet or from supplements. We regularly need two classes of PUFAs, omega-3 and omega-6 fatty acids. In general, the chemical messenger hormones synthesized from omega-6 fatty acids promote (or upregulate) inflammation. Omega-3 fatty acids have the opposite effect: they reduce (or downregulate) inflammation. We need omega-6 and omega-3 essential fatty acids in proper balance to regain balance and FIND HEALTH.

Prior to the development of processed food, humans probably consumed omega-6 and omega-3 fatty acids in approximately equal amounts. But today, most North Americans and Europeans eat far too many omega-6 fatty acids and not enough omega-3 fatty acids, because sources of omega-3 fatty acids have been limited, while sources of omega-6 fatty acids have been abundant (refined vegetable oils, grain-fed animals, and increased meat consumption relative to fish). Furthermore, there is decreased consumption of greens and other vegetable sources of omega-3 fatty acids, and most fast food is rich in omega-6 fatty acids and deficient in omega-3 fatty acids. The unfavorable ratio of omega-6 to omega-3 fatty acids promotes inflammation and may help to explain the rise of asthma, coronary heart disease, many forms of cancer, autoimmunity disorders (such as systemic lupus erythematosis and rheumatoid arthritis), eczema, and neurodegenerative diseases.

Omega-3 Fatty Acids

Omega-3 fatty acids are necessary for physical and mental health. In 2002, the American Heart Association recommended omega-3 fatty acids for patients who had coronary artery disease as long as they obtained their doctor's approval. Omega-3 fatty acids refer to a group of polyunsaturated fatty acids found in certain foods and particularly in fish. Omega-3 fatty acids derived from fish oils are naturally high in both EPA (*eicosapentaenoic acid*) and DHA (*docosahexaenoic acid*). EPA supports heart health. DHA makes up membranes of nerve cells in the brain and is thought to play an important role in normal brain development and function.

Research shows that omega-3 fatty acids may help reduce the risk and symptoms of a variety of disorders. Omega-3 fatty acids can lower triglyceride levels. If your triglycerides are elevated, there is increasing scientific evidence that fish oil and statin drugs are synergistic in their effects on lowering them. Omega-3 fatty acids increase HDL cholesterol (good cholesterol), help minimize inflammation and blood clotting, and keep blood vessels healthy. They help keep the heart beating at a steady rate, and they greatly reduce the risk of sudden cardiac death. They may reduce the risk of getting cancer of the prostate or breast. They may reduce depression. When given to pregnant and nursing mothers, they may increase a baby's IQ, given their impact on brain development.

Sources of omega-3 fatty acids are considerably more limited than for omega-6 fatty acids and include:

→ *Fish*

Good fish sources are oily fish that live in deep, cold water: salmon, mackerel, black cod (sablefish), sardines, herring, and bluefish. However, even leaner, white-fleshed fish provide some omega-3 fatty acids. Consider taking fish oil supplements, which we discuss later in the Add Vitamins/Supplements.

There is concern about the toxic content of fish, particularly too much mercury. In 2004, the FDA and EPA warned women of reproductive age to limit their consumption of some varieties of freshwater fish and some types of ocean fish. The larger the fish, the more mercury and toxin it's going to contain. Mercury can be avoided by eating wild Alaskan salmon (especially sockeye), sardines, herring, and black cod (sablefish).

→ *Walnuts*

About ten percent of the fat in walnuts is omega-3 fatty acid (much higher than in other nuts).

→ *Canola or soybean oil (unhydrogenated)*

→ *Flaxseed*

Whole flaxseeds can be ground fresh and preserved in the refrigerator for up to one week. Preground seeds are more expensive and oxidize rapidly. Flax has a nutty flavor that can complement many foods when added to them. Avoid flaxseed oil, which is expensive, goes rancid easily, and does not contain fiber (flaxseeds have about 3 grams of fiber per tablespoon).

→ *Grass-fed animal fat (rather than grain-fed)*

Omega-6 Fatty Acids

In contrast to omega-3 fatty acids, omega-6 fatty acids are ubiquitous in the American food supply. They build up in the fat of grain-fed animals that we eat. Most snack foods—chips, crackers, cookies, and candy—contain omega-6 fatty acids and no omega-3 fatty acids.

We recommend that you try to balance your intake of omega-3 and omega-6 fatty acids primarily by eating more of the former and less of the latter.

Limiting Fat?

The American Heart Association recommends limiting the amount of fat that you eat each day to twenty-five to thirty-five percent of total calories. For example, that means that if you need 2000 calories per day, total daily fat intake should not exceed 500 – 700 calories. We find it easier to think in terms of grams of fat rather than calories. Remember, there are nine calories per gram of fat, so in this example, total fat consumption would be limited to less than fifty-six to seventy-eight grams of fat.

The American Heart Association also recommends limiting saturated fats to less than seven percent of total daily calories. That means that if you need 2000 calories per day, then no more than 140 of the 2000 calories would come from saturated fat. Again, it may be easier to think in terms of grams of fat. So in eating 2000 calories per day, the total daily saturated fat intake would be less than sixteen grams. Realistically, it isn't possible to eliminate all saturated fat from your diet. Good sources of monounsaturated and polyunsaturated fat also contain small amounts of saturated fat.

There is some controversy regarding limitation of fat intake and consumption of good fats. Some authorities and popular authors recommend that it doesn't matter how much fat is consumed each day as long as the fat is good fat such as olive oil. But respected cardiologist, Dean Ornish, M.D., has demonstrated that regression of coronary artery disease may occur with a very low fat diet. In *The Spectrum*, Dr. Ornish says,

For most people, it's a good idea to reduce total fat consumption. You need only about five percent of calories from fat, or about ten grams per day, to provide the essential fatty acids. The average American eats almost forty percent of calories from fat.

Dr. Ornish goes on to say while good fats are better for you than bad fats, the total amount of fat in your diet is important. All oils are 100 percent fat and fat has nine calories per gram versus four calories per gram for protein and carbohydrates. Therefore, it's easy to eat lots of extra calories if you consume a lot of fat. Olive oil is considered a good fat. However, olive oil contains about fourteen percent saturated fat. One tablespoon of any oil has fourteen grams of fat, which means 126 calories per tablespoon. So one tablespoon of olive oil contains two grams of saturated fat. Dr. Ornish says, "It's not that olive oil lowers your cholesterol. It doesn't raise it as much as bad fat." So, how much good fat should be included in your diet? Dr. Ornish says, "Is olive oil the healthiest fat? In a word, no. It's a better fat, but not the best one."

In October 2006, the FDA authorized new health labeling requirements for canola oil and foods containing canola oil. The labels can say that limited evidence suggests that eating nineteen grams of canola oil daily (that's about one and a half tablespoons) may reduce the risk of heart disease (as long as you also reduce the amount of saturated fat in your diet and don't increase your total caloric intake.) Canola oil is predominantly a monounsaturated fat (good fat) and, as such, is healthier than saturated fats or polyunsaturated oils. However, a wealth of evidence shows that populations that consume good quality olive oil as a primary dietary fat have significantly lower rates of both heart disease and cancer than those that don't. We have no comparable data for canola. Moreover, unlike extra-virgin olive oil, canola oil doesn't contain the antioxidant polyphenols that protect against heart disease and cancer.

Here is our summary of recommendations regarding dietary fat.
- → Replace bad fats with good fats.
- → Avoid *trans* fats (partially hydrogenated and hydrogenated).
- → Eat more omega-3 and less omega-6 fatty acids.
- → Decide how much fat to eat (both total and good fat).

You have to make up your own mind to limit your dietary fat intake—both total and saturated—to or below the recommendations of the American Heart Association and decide how much good fat to eat. If you have risk factors for or already have metabolic syndrome, diabetes, and/or cardiovascular disease, we recommend that you seriously consider doing so.

Eat Healthy Proteins

Most people eat plenty of protein. How much protein is enough? Take in about eight grams of protein for every twenty pounds of body weight. Therefore, a 140-pound woman would need fifty-six grams of protein a day and a 180-pound man would need seventy-two grams.

Regarding protein intake, we recommend that you:

→ eat more vegetable protein: soy foods, other legumes (beans, lentils), whole grains, seeds, and nuts;
→ eat less meat, poultry, and other foods of animal origin; and
→ if you eat fish, select varieties and sources that are likely to have the fewest toxins (refer to previous discussion).

Hydrate

Drink a glass of fluid with meals and between them. Drink plenty of water. Avoid drinking sugared beverages that provide unnecessary empty calories.

Eat More Fiber

Most people do not eat enough dietary fiber, consuming only ten to fifteen grams of fiber per day. For many reasons, including bowel regularity, The American Dietetic Association recommends that people eat twenty-five to thirty-five grams of fiber per day. Most people are five–twenty grams short of that daily goal. Experts urge healthy individuals to add fiber through a well-balanced diet containing high fiber foods (both soluble and insoluble sources of fiber).

Even with a fiber-rich diet, a fiber supplement may be needed to achieve a sufficient fiber intake. Several types of fiber supplements are available. The most natural is a product containing psyllium. Psyllium has the added advantage of lowering cholesterol levels. Although psyllium is generically available, two brand name products that contain psyllium are Metamucil® (3.4 grams per teaspoon) and Konsyl® (6.0 grams per teaspoon). Check the product label to determine the fiber content per serving. Consider adding up to twenty grams of psyllium to your diet each day beginning with three to six grams per day and gradually increasing the amount over several weeks. Be patient; it can take weeks for your gastrointestinal tract to adjust to more fiber. Also be consistent by taking it daily rather than intermittently.

Learn About Nutrition

You now know the fundamentals of nutrition. Eating a healthy diet is essential in maintaining balance and homeostasis. Keep learning. Compare and contrast what you read and hear. The United States Department of Agriculture (USDA) created its well-known Food Guide Pyramid in 1992. Revised in 2010, *My Pyramid*, while well-intended, does not go far enough to clearly guide Americans on how to stay healthy because of strong influence of the food industry on U.S. food policy. There are better resources out there amid the myriad of diet books available. Here are three recommendations.

Walter Willett, M.D. is Professor of Epidemiology and Nutrition, chairman of the Department of Nutrition at Harvard School of Public Health, and professor of medicine at Harvard Medical School. He is the world's leading authority on nutrition. Mollie Katzen is listed by *The New York Times* as one of the best-selling cookbook authors of all time. In their book, *Eat, Drink, and Weigh Less*, they argue, "MyPyramid is riddled with misguided recommendations that ignore evidence about health and diet collected over the last forty years." Their pyramid is "...a more useful, informative, and accurate alternative."

We agree and also encourage you to take a look at *The South Beach Diet* by Dr. Arthur Agatston. A firm believer in the education and empowerment of his patients and the public at large, his books and Internet site are valuable resources for healthy lifestyle and disease prevention information.

A third resource is the world-renowned leader and pioneer of integrative medicine, Dr. Andrew Weil. His *Anti-Inflammatory Diet and Food Pyramid* is available on his Internet site and in his publications. Dr. Weil maintains that following an anti-inflammatory diet reduces chronic inflammation that underlies many serious diseases that become more common as people age. On his Internet site, he says, "It is a way of selecting and preparing foods based on science that can help people achieve and maintain optimum health over their lifetime." We agree.

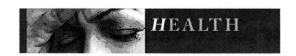

Hold YOUR Weight Down and Watch Your Waist

Perhaps you have calculated your BMI so that you could determine your daily caloric needs. Now you get to find out where all of those extra calories you may be eating have likely gone. Look down. You guessed it: your belly!

WATCH BOTH YOUR WEIGHT AND WAIST

By measuring your waist circumference, you can see if you have abnormal belly fat. If you do, you either have or are at risk for developing metabolic syndrome (also known as metabolic syndrome X and insulin resistance). Arthur Agatston, M.D., author of the *South Beach Diet* books, reinforces this point. In *The South Beach Heart Health Revolution,* he states that:

"There is an important medical condition so obvious that I can diagnose it without performing a single diagnostic test."

Dr. Agatston is talking about metabolic syndrome. He goes on to write, "It has reached epidemic proportions in the United States." You can appreciate why he is concerned because you now understand the interrelationships of medically unexplained symptoms and metabolic syndrome. The former are not life threatening. The latter can kill you, and you're the only one who can prevent or cure the condition. After the age of forty, a man has about a fifty percent risk of developing coronary artery disease at some point in his life. Heart disease is the number one cause of death in women. Steven Nissen is the chairman of the department of cardiovascular medicine at the Cleveland Clinic, considered one of the finest heart centers in the world. In a 2007 article in *Best Life,* he is quoted as saying,

"METABOLIC SYNDROME IS THE DISEASE OF THE NEW MILLENNIUM"

People with a cluster of metabolic syndrome symptoms have a disproportionate risk for heart disease as well as diabetes and stroke.

What is this cluster of metabolic syndrome symptoms? It is:

→ Hypertension: high blood pressure of 130/85 or above, but in general, any elevation above 115/75 increases cardiovascular risk;

→ Hyperglycemia: fasting blood sugar equal to or more than 110 mg/dL or evidence of prediabetes;

→ High triglycerides in the blood: blood fats that promote plaque buildup in the arteries;

→ Low levels of HDL (good) cholesterol; and elevated levels of LDL (bad) cholesterol, which raise the risk of heart and vascular disease;

→ Excess abdominal weight (fat): waistline greater than forty inches for men and thirty-five for women (but any increase in your waistline over normal may confer risk);

→ Fatty liver (detected by elevated liver blood tests and/or on liver scan with ultrasound or CT); and

→ BMI > 30: central obesity can be assumed if the BMI is this high.

The epidemic of metabolic syndrome has spread to adolescents and young adults.

Studies now show that ten percent of high school graduating seniors have metabolic syndrome. The problem creeps up on you as you age, beginning with a few extra pounds and an increase in blood pressure. It slowly progresses until you are diagnosed with metabolic syndrome, which can lead to diabetes, heart attack, and stroke. According to the National Institutes of Health, seventy-five million Americans have metabolic syndrome. This is part of the epidemic we've alerted you to.

FAT AROUND THE MIDDLE OF YOUR BODY IS DANGEROUS

It acts like an endocrine organ in the body—like a gland secreting harmful stuff—producing biologically active molecules, which cause chronic low grade inflammation and increase the risk for metabolic syndrome insulin resistance. Insulin is made by the pancreas and allows the body to process blood sugar, or glucose. Insulin is also responsible for sending excess glucose to the liver where it is stored as glycogen for later use. Insulin sensitivity is the measure of how well your body uses glucose for energy.

The higher your sensitivity, the more efficiently your body uses glucose and the lower your diabetes risk. The problem begins with central body fat whether you are overweight or obese or not. This fat manifests symptomatically as an enlarged waistline and is deposited not only in your abdominal wall (subcutaneous fat, which is the stuff you can actually grab), but more importantly, within the abdomen (visceral fat within your torso). This visceral abdominal fat causes chronic inflammation and impairs insulin sensitivity. Consequently, blood sugar spikes and the pancreas produces extra insulin, which can lead to type-2 diabetes.

While belly fat can affect your entire body adversely, it frequently involves the liver.

Fatty liver is the most common cause of liver blood test abnormalities. While excess alcohol intake can cause fatty liver, the most common cause by far is what is called non-alcoholic fatty liver disease or NAFLD. Most of the time, the fat does not damage the liver. However, in approximately ten percent of people with fatty liver, the fat becomes associated with inflammation. This is called *non-alcoholic steato hepatitis* (NASH). *Steato* means fat and *hepatitis* means inflammation. Some people with NASH develop cirrhosis, which occurs when liver tissue is replaced by scar tissue. Complications from cirrhosis can be fatal.

MEASURE YOUR WAIST CIRCUMFERENCE

Use a measuring tape to measure your waist at the level of your belly button. As a rule of thumb for any age and sex, your waist circumference should be less than one-half of your height. Current U.S. guidelines define normal waist circumference as less than thirty-one inches in women and thirty-seven inches in men, and elevated waist circumference as more than thirty-five inches in women and forty inches in men. The middle zone of marginally elevated values has been considered a gray area largely disregarded by doctors and researchers. Science now shows that waist circumference is a continuous risk factor.

Most people don't realize that they can have belly fat and metabolic syndrome even if they aren't overweight.

There is risk when the waist size is greater than thirty-one inches in women and thirty-seven inches in men. Mayo Clinic research presented at the American College of Cardiology's Annual Scientific Session in Chicago, April 2008, shows that more than one-half of American adults considered to have a normal body weight have high body fat percentages— greater than twenty percent for men and thirty percent for women—as well as heart and metabolic disturbances. The research confirmed that those with the highest percentage of body fat were also those who had metabolic disturbances linked to heart disease. The Mayo Clinic researchers call this *normal weight obesity*. They define normal weight obesity as a condition of having a normal BMI with high body fat percentage. "Using the term 'normal weight obesity' is really a way of being more precise about the changing conceptualization of obesity, because the real definition of obesity is excess body fat," says Francisco Lopez-Jimenez, M.D., a cardiologist on the Mayo research team. He adds,

"Our study demonstrates that even people with normal weight may have excessive body fat, and that these people are at risk for metabolic abnormalities that lead to diabetes and, eventually, to heart disease."

One of the authors has had personal experience with this.

THE AUTHOR'S PERSONAL HISTORY OF NORMAL WEIGHT OBESITY

I (WBS) found out the hard way that I had normal weight obesity when I was diagnosed with coronary artery disease. You may want to re-read my case presentation in Chapter 4.

"You probably have a form of metabolic syndrome."

After shocking me with the diagnosis of coronary artery disease, Dr. John Rumberger told me I had an abnormal amount of belly fat. I thought,

First you find out you have heart disease. Now you find out that you have too much fat in your belly!

I had normal weight obesity, which is a risk factor for metabolic syndrome. When I was diagnosed, I was twenty-five pounds heavier than in high school with an extra four inches around my waist. Assembling my risk factors for metabolic syndrome, I include (not necessarily in order of importance):

→ Normal weight obesity;
→ LDL (bad) cholesterol, too high for me (it was 120 mg/dL);

Technically, LDL is not part of the metabolic syndrome, but it plays a very important role in the development of atherosclerosis;

→ Family history;

Both of my parents have late-life vascular problems. They are in their late 80s, and both are hypertensive, have excess belly fat, and my mother just recovered from a stroke;

↦ Intermittent mild hypertension; and

↦ Stress.

I personally suspect that stress was my biggest risk factor.

I hope my story helps convince you to assess yourself accurately and take responsibility for your health. Your health is too important to waist away.

TRY TO LOSE AT LEAST TEN PERCENT
OF YOUR EXCESS WEIGHT

Since we also advocate resistance training, you can weigh more if the extra that you carry is mainly muscle. Even if you can lose ten only percent of your excess weight, most of it will come off your belly.

You can reduce your risks of metabolic syndrome by losing weight.

Recall your study of the harmful effects of stress. Weight loss not only reduces the stress of oxidation and inflammation, it improves each of the components of the cluster list of metabolic syndrome (review the list at the beginning of the chapter). A new study published in the December 14-28, 2009 issue of the *Archives of Internal Medicine* reports that men who stay slim, active, and smoke free have a fifty-nine percent lower risk of coronary heart disease events and seventy-seven percent lower risk of dying of cardiovascular disease.

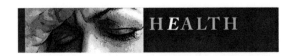

Exercise Regularly

You have already learned about the benefits of exercise on the mind/ brain. Furthermore, your level of physical activity is the single most important factor that predicts whether, as you age, you will feel and look weak and unhealthy and whether you will become frail and susceptible to falling. Human beings are designed to be physically active. Frailty is not inevitable. The maintenance of physical activity throughout your life is related to the emergence of your health. This was one of the strongest correlations found in the MacArthur Foundation's 1998 study of aging in America as reported in the book *Successful Aging*. Staying physically active affects all of your mind/brain systems.

Exercise helps reduce and eliminate symptoms, reduce the stress response, elevate mood and positive emotions, and promote positive thinking and self-control.

It's time for you to get moving.

HOW MUCH EXERCISE?

The consensus on recommendations for physical activity is a minimum of thirty minutes of moderate intensity activity on most days of the week, or 150 minutes per week. There is a growing consensus that more exercise may be necessary to enhance long-term weight loss. The American College of Sports Medicine and the American Heart Association have jointly developed exercise guidelines that are available on the Internet (see **Bibliography**). All healthy adults between the ages of eighteen to sixty-five should be getting at least thirty minutes of moderate intensity activity five days of the week. However, there are additional guidelines for those sixty-five and older or for those fifty to sixty-four with chronic conditions or physical functional limitations (e.g., arthritis) that affect movement ability or physical fitness.

TYPES OF EXERCISE

There are three components to exercise: aerobics, resistance or strength training, and flexibility/balance.

Aerobics (Cardio Conditioning)

For exercise and health, the Surgeon General's recommendation for physical activity is to add at least thirty minutes of moderately intense physical activity on top of your customary daily activities. This exercise strengthens your heart and helps you gain the stamina and endurance to live a healthy life from day to day.

The best way to start exercising is to walk.

Walking for Fitness

Walk for a minimum of thirty minutes each day. This can be broken up into shorter periods—say three ten-minute walks—in order to achieve the goal. If you have been inactive, walk as far as you can without feeling fatigued or stressed, even if you can only last for a few minutes. Then, gradually increase your walking time until you can walk briskly for at least thirty minutes without discomfort. If you have been active, you can move directly to the thirty-minute or longer brisk walk.

What does the term *brisk* mean? We recommend the method described by Dr. Agatston in *The South Beach Heart Health Revolution*. Think of a scale from one to ten with one being the slowest possible walking speed and ten being the fastest that you can walk without getting out of breath. Walking briskly is going at a pace of six to seven, which means that you're working moderately hard. Try to work up a light sweat, which is another indication that you are working hard enough. Start your walk with a five-minute warm-up at an intensity level of three to four for the first three to four minutes and work up to a pace of six to seven during the final minute. Take a twenty-minute walk at this pace and go longer if you want more exercise. Then, cool down over five minutes by reducing your speed to a level of three to four again. Take several deep breaths before you stop, which will help relax and invigorate you. As your fitness improves, you will be able to increase the intensity of your workout to the eight to ten ranges. You do not want to be out of breath at ten, and you should be able to carry on a conversation.

Another approach to measure the intensity of your exercise more accurately is to use your target heart rate to determine your correct level of exertion. Either purchase a fitness monitor or learn how to take your own pulse rate and exercise at least sixty percent of your maximum heart rate (which varies based upon age). You can exercise harder with higher heart rate and derive even greater fitness benefits. However, you should probably consult with your doctor and/or fitness professional before exercising significantly above sixty percent of maximum heart rate.

Walking for Weight Management

For weight management, studies now show that the goal is to take 10,000 steps each day. You may take anywhere from 900 to 3,000 steps during an ordinary day, so you can see that unless you have an unusually physical job, you will need to take an intentional walk. Taking 10,000 steps is the approximate equivalent of walking five miles. The actual distance covered depends upon the length of your stride. Consider purchasing a pedometer. The average person will burn 100 calories by walking a mile, so walking five miles burns approximately 500 calories.

Alternatives to Walking

You can substitute other exercises such as bicycling, swimming, or stair climbing to burn an equivalent number of calories to walking. You will need to determine how long to exercise to burn 500 calories. The United States government has an Internet calculator called the Physical Activity Calculator, which is referenced in the **Bibliography**. This calculator will permit you to determine the calories expended for a physical activity, depending not only on the type of activity, but also on your weight. It takes more energy (calories) to move more weight.

Strength (Resistance) Training

Without engaging in resistance training, most adults lose muscle and gain fat as they age. Between the ages of twenty and fifty, the average person loses one-half pound of muscle per year and replaces it with up to one and one-half pounds of fat. Muscle declines with age as it is replaced with fat. Without resistance exercise, even if a twenty-year-old person turns fifty without having gained any weight—highly unlikely these days—he or she would have replaced fifteen pounds of muscle with fat. Can you see how easily you can develop normal weight obesity? The reality for most of us is that we also gain additional weight attributed to fat accumulation.

When we lose muscle, we lose life function. The most important risk of loss of muscular function as we age is the increased risk of falling.

If you do not have experience with strength training, we recommend that you begin slowly and work with a qualified personal trainer or instructor in an exercise facility. It is important to use resistance equipment correctly to minimize risk of injury and maximize benefits. You can decide later whether to continue working with a professional, work out on your own at the gym, and/or at home with your own equipment.

Experts recommend a minimum of eight-ten strength training exercises involving the major muscle groups, each with eight-twelve repetitions performed twice a week. To get you started, we recommend five strength-training exercises that you can do on your own without equipment. They exercise the legs, core, and upper body. These compound exercises will strengthen your most important muscle groups. The term compound means that several major muscle groups are being exercised. You don't need special equipment to do these exercises.

Legs

As you age, weakness of your legs, particularly your thighs, increases your chance of falling. Here's how to strengthen them.

Squats

Stand with your feet slightly wider than shoulder-width apart and with your hands by your side. Keeping your back straight, squat down to the point where your thighs are approximately parallel to the floor (or before, if you have pain in your knees or lower back). You can have a chair under your bottom for security if you prefer. Pause, and then rise to the original standing position. Keep your gaze forward. Breathe in on the way down and breathe out on the way up. When twelve repetitions become easy, you can add resistance by holding dumbbells or other weighted objects at your sides.

Lunges

Stand with your feet shoulder-width apart and your hands on your hips. Step forward with one of your feet, bending at the knee so that the thigh is parallel to the floor (or before, if you have pain in your knees or lover back). Make sure that your knee does not extend farther than your foot. Pause, then step back into the original standing position. Repeat with the other foot. Breathe in when you lunge forward and breathe out when you step back. When twelve repetitions become easy, you can add resistance by holding dumbbells or other weighted objects at your sides.

Core

Having a strong mid-section or core supports your back muscles and reduces your risk of injury. Here are two exercises directed to core strength.

Abdominal crunches

Lie on your back with your knees bent and feet flat on the floor. Put your hands lightly to your ears. Crunch up about thirty degrees from the floor by using your abdominal muscles.

Arm and leg lifts

Place both hands and knees on the floor with your arms and thighs parallel to each other and perpendicular to the floor. Make sure that your knees are directly under your hips. Your hands should be under your shoulders. Looking at the floor, keep your head in line with your spine and back straight. Lift one arm and the opposite leg slowly off the floor and extend them straight out so that your leg, back, and arm are roughly in one line. Slowly lower them to the starting position. After one set, switch positions and use the other arm and leg in opposition.

Upper Body

The classic push-up is the single best exercise you can do for the upper body without special equipment.

Push-ups

Get into the classic push-up position with your hands on the floor at shoulder-width apart. Keep your back straight and your toes or knees on the floor. Lower yourself until your chest almost touches the floor and then push back up. If you don't have the necessary strength, you can modify the push-up by keeping your knees on the ground. When they become easy, you can increase the number of repetitions.

Flexibility and Balance

Include at least five minutes of stretching and balancing each day, preferably after you walk or do an alternative exercise. Yoga includes stretching, balance, and strength training. It is a mind, body, and soul activity. We suggest that you begin your program by learning the yoga sun salutation. You can add to or replace this with flexibility and balancing exercises that you choose for your personal plan.

Step 1:

Stand (facing the direction of the sun) with both feet touching. Bring the hands together, palm-to-palm, at the heart. Exhale.

Step 2:

Inhale and raise the arms slowly upward. Slowly bend backward, stretching arms above the head.

Step 3:

Exhale while you slowly bend forward until your hands are in line with your feet, touching your head to your knees (if possible). Press your palms down, fingertips in line with toes (bend your knees if necessary), and touch the floor.

Step 4:

Inhale and move the right leg back away from the body in a wide backward step. Keep your hands and feet firmly on the ground with the left foot between the hands. Raise your head.

Step 5:

While exhaling, bring the left foot together with the right. Keep arms straight, raise the hips, and align the head with the arms, forming an upward arch.

Step 6:

Exhale and lower the body to the floor until the feet, knees, hands, chest, and forehead touch the ground.

Step 7:

Inhale and slowly raise the head and bend backward as much as possible, bending the spine to the maximum.

Step 8:

While exhaling, bring the left foot together with the right. Keep arms straight, raise the hips, and align the head with the arms, forming an upward arch.

Step 9:

Inhale and move the right leg back from the body in a wide backward step. Keep the hands and feet firmly on the ground with the left foot between the hands. Raise the head.

Step 10:

Exhale while you slowly bend forward until your hands are in line with your feet, touching your head to your knees (if possible). Press your palms down, fingertips in line with toes (bend your knees if necessary), and touch the floor.

Step 11:

Inhale and raise the arms slowly upward. Slowly bend backward, stretching arms above the head. Inhale.

Step 12:

Stand (facing the direction of the sun) with both feet touching. Bring the hands together, palm-to-palm, at the heart. Exhale.

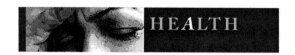

Add Vitamins/Supplements

One of our friends, Denny Walsh, says, "You're healthy as long as your vitamins outnumber your medications." While that's not always possible, it seems to us to be a good goal, especially since the risk of developing metabolic syndrome can be greatly reduced with the lifestyle changes advocated in **PART 4** of this book. Eating a healthy diet is of primary importance, but you should also take a daily multivitamin and consider taking several supplements. Take care and take time to check out thoroughly what supplements and multivitamin are right for you. As you consider adding them to your dietary intake, consult with your doctor and/or pharmacist to maintain balanced use of these products. Your health depends on it. We offer you some guidelines here.

TAKE A MULTIVITAMIN DAILY

Most people don't get enough vitamins and minerals in their diets, so the dollar that you spend on this each day will be worthwhile. Note that Harvard's Dr. Walter Willett, Dr. Andrew Weil, and many other authorities on health advocate the health insurance of taking a daily multivitamin. Remember, a multivitamin is in addition to a healthy diet and not a replacement for one.

Taking a multivitamin is not a license to eat poorly. What you include in your diet is as important as what you exclude. There are at least 1,000 protective substances that are found in certain foods. Many have anti-cancer, anti-aging, and anti-heart disease properties. They are found mainly in vegetables, fruits, whole grains, legumes, and soy products. The pigments that account for the various colors of vegetables and fruits have antioxidant properties that confer protection against cancer and other chronic diseases, as well as protection from a range of environmental toxins, including pesticides. Eat every day from as many parts of the color spectrum as you can.

We recommend that your multivitamin contain what we have listed below, and as are described by Andrew Weil, M.D. in his book *Healthy Aging* and on his Internet site. A good multivitamin with these components will probably include more than one pill or capsule. It (they) can be taken at any time of the day and after eating to avoid indigestion and nausea. Vitamin D, vitamin E, and carotenoids require some fat to be absorbed. So you might not get absorption of these components if you take the multivitamin after eating a low-fat or no fat breakfast.

Vitamin A

Look for a mixture of antioxidant carotenoids, which includes beta-carotene, alpha-carotene, lutein, and lycopene. These are labeled collectively as "mixed carotenoids," or "provitamin A." The body converts these antioxidants that are found in fruits and vegetables into usable retinoids. Find a daily vitamin with 10,000 to 15,000 IU of mixed carotenoids including beta-carotene. If you are a smoker, be aware that taking more than 30,000 IU of beta-carotene daily may increase the risk of lung cancer. Avoid multivitamin products containing preformed vitamin A, which is often listed as retinol or as vitamin A palmitate or acetate.

B Vitamins

Your multivitamin should include 50 mg each of most B vitamins, with the exception of folic acid (at least 400 mcg) and vitamin B12, whose chemical name is cyanocobalamin (at least 50 mcg).

If you are a woman and are at risk for age-related macular degeneration, consider taking daily supplementation with folic acid (2.5 mg), pyridoxine hydrochloride (50 mg), and vitamin B12 (1 mg or 1000 micrograms), since a recent study published in the *Archives of Internal Medicine* found that doing so may reduce this risk.

Vitamin C

Take at least 60 mg of this antioxidant daily and optimally 200 to 250 mg for optimum health (this is all that the body can use in a day). If your multivitamin only includes 60 mg of vitamin C, then take an additional 200 mg. Don't pay extra for "natural" vitamin C, since there is no difference in effectiveness or absorption between natural and synthetic L-ascorbic acid (the chemical name of vitamin C).

Vitamin D

We recommend that you take at least 1,000 to 2,000 IU of vitamin D each day. Most multivitamins contain only 400 IU. There are two forms: D2 (ergocalciferol), which is created during plant photosynthesis, and D3 (cholecalciferol), which is made when human skin is exposed to the UVB rays from sunlight. The best form to take is D3, since it is the form that your body creates naturally and is better absorbed and utilized.

Vitamin E

This is a complex group including four tocopherols and four tocotrienols known as alpha, beta, gamma, and delta for both. Take a multivitamin that preferably has 80 mg of mixed natural tocopherols and tocotrienols (with at least 10 mg of tocotrienols). An alternative is to take a multivitamin with 400 IU of mixed natural tocopherols a day. Avoid products with synthetic dl-alpha-tocopherol or d-alpha-tocopherol.

Iron

The multivitamin should not contain iron unless you have been diagnosed with iron deficiency anemia, since this mineral facilitates oxidation and may increase the risk of heart disease and cancer.

Selenium

Take no more than 200 mcg daily.

Vitamin K

There are two forms: K1 (phylloquinone), which is produced by plants, and K2 (menaquinones) formed from K1 by bacteria in the digestive tract or obtained from certain foods. Most people should take a multivitamin that contains vitamin K. If you have osteoporosis or osteopenia, take 50 to 100 mcg of vitamin K daily and be aware that most multivitamins contain less.

TAKE 3 GRAMS OF FISH OIL SUPPLEMENTS DAILY

After a multivitamin, the second most important supplement for most people to take each day is fish oil, which contains important omega-3 fatty acids that were discussed in Dine Well. EPA (eicosapentaenoic acid) seems to have heart protective effects and DHA (docosahexaenoic acid) seems to be of benefit to the nervous system. Consider taking two to three grams (2,000 to 3,000 mg) of fish oil that contains both EPA and DHA. Be sure that you read the label and add the contents of DHA and EPA together to determine how much is contained in each capsule, because you want to take a total of two to three grams each day. Prescription forms of omega-3 fatty acids are also available.

Purchase a brand that is distilled and certified to be free of mercury and other toxins. According to a July 2003 survey conducted by *Consumer Reports*, all of the top sixteen brands of fish oil have been verified to have the same high quality and purity of EPA and DHA as described on the label. *Consumer Reports* recommends that you shop by price. Don't use cod liver oil because many brands contain too much vitamin A. Flaxseed oil doesn't seem to have the same therapeutic effects of fish oil.

TAKE 1,000 TO 2,000 IU VITAMIN D AS A SUPPLEMENT DAILY

Fifty percent of Americans are deficient in vitamin D. Vitamin D deficiency is a risk factor for the development of weak bones and fractures related to osteomalacia (which is often mistaken for osteoporosis). New scientific studies confirm the importance of vitamin D for health.

There are vitamin D receptors on the cells throughout the body. By controlling more than 200 genes, vitamin D may reduce the risk of many chronic illnesses including cancer of the colon, prostate, and breast; autoimmune diseases such as multiple sclerosis and Crohn's disease; diabetes, and cardiovascular disease.

Obesity increases risk for vitamin D deficiency. Studies also show an inverse association between vitamin D status and diabetes and the metabolic syndrome.

Sensible sun exposure can provide adequate vitamin D during the summer months, but dermatologists do not recommend sun exposure. This would require the exposure of one's arms and legs without sunscreen for 5-30 minutes depending upon the time of day, season, and skin pigmentation. The face should be protected since the sun can cause wrinkles and some skin cancers. Sunburn should be avoided. Melanoma is most closely linked to burns.

FORTIFY YOUR DIET WITH DAILY CALCIUM AND MAGNESIUM SUPPLEMENTS

Two minerals are particularly important in your diet: calcium and magnesium.

Calcium

Calcium is the most abundant mineral in the body. It is present mainly in the bones and teeth. Calcium is an essential dietary element that is necessary for good bone health, efficient nerve and muscle function, and overall cardiovascular health. It may help prevent cancers of the digestive tract. It is associated with relieving mood swings and food cravings and reducing the pain, tenderness, and bloating associated with premenstrual syndrome. Your bones serve as a storage site for the body's calcium by providing this mineral to the bloodstream for use by the heart and other organs. Eating a diet rich in calcium helps to restore it to the bones. Supplements can help as well. Men should take 1,000 to 1,200 milligrams of calcium a day; women under sixty should take about 1,200 of calcium a day. Women over sixty should take 1,600 milligrams of calcium each day. Since most of us cannot absorb more than 600 milligrams of calcium at a time, it is best to divide the daily dose in two and take it twice a day.

Magnesium

Magnesium is an essential element that is needed for proper functioning of the nervous, muscular, and cardiovascular systems. Consider taking half as much magnesium as calcium. Magnesium can offset the constipating effect of calcium and assure that there is an appropriate balance of these two key elements in the body. Take magnesium citrate, chelate, or glycinate, since magnesium oxide can irritate the digestive tract, resulting in a laxative effect and diarrhea.

GIVE THOUGHT TO TAKING AT LEAST 400 MG OF PLANT STEROLS (PHYTOSTEROLS) TWICE A DAY

The United States Food and Drug Administration (FDA) has determined that foods and/or supplements containing at least 0.4 g (400 mg.) per serving of plant sterols (also called *phytosterols*), when taken twice a day with meals as part of a low saturated fat, low trans fat, and low cholesterol diet, may reduce the risk of heart disease. Cardiovascular disease remains the number one cause of death for both men and women in the United States. Elevated levels of bad LDL cholesterol are generally recognized as a major risk factor for heart disease. Diet and lifestyle modification are very important but often do not provide sufficient reductions. While a variety of medications are available to treat cardiovascular disease, plant sterols are natural alternatives.

Just as the animal sterol cholesterol is present in all animal species, plant sterols are found in all plants. The best dietary sources of plant sterols are vegetables, seeds, and nuts. Plant sterols are a class of fat-like plant compounds with chemical structures similar to cholesterol. Clinical evidence over the past fifty years has consistently demonstrated that consumption of plant sterols inhibits the intestinal absorption of cholesterol and produces decreases in LDL cholesterol from eight to fifteen percent. There are no reported serious side effects or adverse reactions. Plant sterols have been added to a variety of food products worldwide with no adverse impact on taste or texture. Foods containing added plant sterols such as orange juice, margarine, butter spreads, mayonnaise, milk, yogurt, cheese, and dairy substitutes are advertised and labeled as potentially lowering or removing cholesterol. Plant sterols can be found in supplement form and in combination with aspirin.

CONSIDER TAKING A DAILY ASPIRIN TO PREVENT HEART ATTACK (AFTER CHECKING WITH YOUR DOCTOR)

Taking a daily aspirin can reduce the risk of heart attack by up to thirty percent. Based on the available evidence, the American Heart Association and the U.S. Preventive Services Task Force recommend that doctors consider aspirin therapy for the prevention of a first heart attack in individuals identified to be at increased risk for cardiovascular events.

HERBS

Herbs can be as powerful as prescription drugs. Twenty-five percent of all pharmaceutical drugs are derivatives of trees, shrubs, or herbs. Thus, it is important to be certain that any natural product you decide to take is safe and does not interfere with prescribed drugs. Be sure that your doctor knows everything that you are taking.

"NATURAL"

"Natural" does not necessarily equate with safe. In 1994, Congress passed the Dietary Supplement Health and Education Act. Vitamins, minerals, herbs, and other natural substances on store shelves do not require review or approval from the Food and Drug Administration. As part of this law, supplement manufacturers were advised that they were required to substantiate the safety of their ingredients. However, this has not been enforced until recently. The FDA phased in the requirement that supplement manufacturers test the purity and composition of their products, and companies have a deadline date to comply. Even more regulation is likely to be enacted soon.

PROBIOTICS

Considerable scientific research is now being directed to the health benefits of probiotics, which are dietary substances containing potentially beneficial bacteria or yeasts. The official definition of probiotics is, *Live microorganisms which, when administered in adequate amounts, confer a health benefit on the host.* According to Lynne V. McFarland, Ph.D. of the Veterans Affairs Puget Sound Healthcare System, when speaking at the International Probiotic Association World Congress in 2008, "The Food and Drug Administration provides little regulation of probiotic products, and products available to the consumer vary greatly in quality and the level of evidence supporting their label claims." She goes on to say,

When the consumers go in and they want to buy their own probiotic . . . it's chaos. There are so many different probiotic products out on the market, and the diversity of quality can be all the way from fine pharmaceutical manufacturers to [someone who makes it] in his bathtub.

CONSIDER TAKING ADDITIONAL ANTIOXIDANT SUPPORT

In addition to the antioxidants that you get from your diet and multivitamin, you can consider taking two additional supplements that have the most scientific support.

Co-Q-10

Co-Q-10 (ubiquinone) is an antioxidant made by the body that increases oxygen use by the cell. Consider taking it if you are at risk for or already have metabolic syndrome or if you have a susceptible family history. The dose is thirty milligrams per day, which must be taken with some fat to be absorbed. Consider taking Co-Q-10 if you are taking a statin drug, which can inhibit the body's own production. Co-Q-10 is now commonly included in some better quality multivitamins, so check the label.

Alpha Lipoic Acid with Acetyl-L-Carnitine

Here's another regimen to consider relative to metabolic syndrome. There is evidence that the combination of alpha lipoic acid (ALA) and acetyl-l-carnitine (ALC) may slow the cell aging process. They are used in the mitochondria, which are the cell's energy center. ALA and ALC may reduce insulin resistance and augment the body's antioxidant defenses.

The constituents can be purchased individually or combined as a product called Juvenon™. The recommended dosage is 400 mg of ALA and 1,000 mg of ALC taken daily with food.

CONSIDER ADDITIONAL ANTI-INFLAMMATORY SUPPORT

In addition to eating an anti-inflammatory diet, you can consider taking anti-inflammatory supplements.

Turmeric and Ginger

Turmeric is the yellow spice in American mustard and Indian curries. Curcumin is one of turmeric's components. It has powerful antioxidant properties and may protect against the development of Alzheimer's disease, which is associated with brain inflammation. It also has broad anti-inflammatory and anti-cancer effects. Turmeric is available as a tea or supplement.

Ginger also has anti-inflammatory effects. It is available as a tea, candy, or supplement.

GET ADEQUATE SLEEP

Science has confirmed that sleep deprivation is bad for your health. The most remarkable studies show that the less people sleep, the more likely they are to become obese, which predisposes them to development of metabolic syndrome. Sleep deprivation may also increase levels of stress hormones, raise blood pressure, contribute to allostatic load (bad stress), and increase levels of chemical transmitters responsible for increasing inflammation.

Most people do not get enough sleep and many suffer from insomnia. The National Institute of Health recommends that adults need seven hours to nine hours of sleep nightly. With this goal in mind, avoid taking alcohol and caffeine within three to four hours of bedtime. If necessary, you can consider two natural sleep aids, valerian and/or melatonin.

Valerian

Valerian is an herb that has been used as a sedative for centuries. Standardized extracts are available in health food and grocery stores and pharmacies. Take one to two capsules a half hour before bedtime.

Melatonin

Melatonin is a hormone naturally found in the body that regulates the sleep/wake cycle and other daily biorhythms. Consider taking tablets that dissolve after being placed under the tongue. After ensuring that your bedroom is completely dark, take 2.5 mg at bedtime as an occasional dose. If regular use is preferred, take a much lower dose, 0.25 to 0.3 mg.

CONSIDER AVOIDING NICOTINE AND CAFFEINE; IF YOU DRINK ALCOHOL, DO SO IN MODERATION

While this chapter has discussed additions, here's our advice on subtractions. While smoking is obviously to be avoided because it is unhealthy and contributes to allostatic load (bad stress), understand that both nicotine and caffeine are sympathomimetic substances. Recall that the sympathetic nervous system of the autonomic nervous system plays a critical role in the stress response and can contribute to the generation and perpetuation of chronic pain and symptoms. Caffeine and nicotine activate the sympathetic nervous system, so you may want to try avoiding them to see if anxiety decreases and/or symptoms improve.

Moderate alcohol consumption may provide some health benefits, including reducing the risk of developing heart disease and peripheral vascular disease. However, anything more than moderate drinking can cancel potential benefits and result in serious health problems. Moderate drinking is defined as two drinks a day if you're a male sixty-five and younger or one drink a day if you're a female or a male sixty-six and older. A drink is defined as twelve ounces (355 milliliters) of beer, five ounces (148 milliliters) of wine or 1.5 ounces (44 milliliters) of 80-proof distilled spirits.

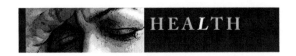

Learn How Doctors Think
and How to Work with Them

E veryone hurts.

You know how to see behind your symptoms, but you still need professional help at times. Jerome Groopman, M.D. is a Harvard hematologist/ oncologist and medical author. He has something very important to tell you about your health,

"The state of medical care is that there is going to be less and less time to do an imperfect science."

Life is too fast, and the hurry affects your relationship with doctors and other care professionals. Moreover, medical science doesn't have all of the answers. Doctors vary in how much time they will spend with you and how much knowledge, skill, and art they possess.

What is the "art of medicine?"

Cardiologist Bernadine Healy, M.D. is the former head of both the National Institutes of Health and the American Red Cross. She is a senior writer for *U.S. News & World Report*. In the July 14, 2007 issue, she says: "Before you dismiss this notion of 'art' as squishy or outmoded, understand what it means. As old as the ancient temples and as contemporary as the decoded genome, it can be summed up in four principles: Mastery. Individuality. Humanity. Morality." While most doctors are well meaning, some are not artists. In the healing arts, we have forgotten where we came from. And in our forgetfulness, we have neglected holistic care. A front-page article by Jacob Goldstein in the April 29, 2008 issue of *The Wall Street Journal* says,

To adapt, American medicine is drifting away from the old standard—in which a single doctor handled almost all of a patient's needs—and toward a more team-based approach. This system includes not only multiple doctors but also nurse practitioners and physician assistants.

Your care increasingly involves multiple professionals. Unfortunately, you have learned how fragmented and disintegrated the system has become. This is particularly apparent when practitioners try to deal with medically unexplained symptoms and syndromes.

Furthermore, there is the problem of *medicalization*. Remember the question from Chapter 1 that medical sociologist Peter Conrad asks in *The Medicalization of Society: On the Transformation of Human Conditions into Treatable Disorders*. It has to do with the multiple illnesses, syndromes, psychological states, and behavior that now receive medical diagnosis and medical treatment. He asks,

"Does it mean that a whole range of life's problems have now received medical diagnoses and are subject to medical treatment, despite dubious evidence of their medical nature?"

Health columnist Tara Parker-Pope writes in July 29, 2008 issue of *The New York Times*,

"A growing chorus of discontent suggests that the once-revered doctor-patient relationship is on the rocks."

She goes on to say the relationship is the cornerstone of the medical system and that if patients and doctors aren't getting along, nobody can be helped. She adds,

"But increasingly, research and anecdotal reports suggest that many patients don't trust doctors."

THIS ISN'T GOOD!

Dr. Groopman's *How Doctors Think* deserves your attention. Christine Gorman of *Time* magazine calls it, "Must reading for every physician who cares for patients and every patient who wishes to get the best care"; and William Grimes of *The New York Times* writes, "This is medicine at its best, 'a mix of science and soul'."The point of Dr. Groopman's book is that for you to assume responsibility for your own health, you need to understand what's really going on with doctors and the medical system. That's our point, too.

It's time for a reality check here. Let's review from Chapter 1.

A SUMMARY OF WHAT'S GOING ON IN THE WORLD OF MODERN HEALTH CARE

→ Everyone hurts.

→ Time with doctors is increasingly limited.

→ Medical science is imperfect.

→ Medicine is both art and science.

→ Few understand that the whole is greater than the sum of its parts.

→ Care of the person is increasingly fragmented from within (with multiple symptoms that are seemingly unrelated) and without (multiple doctors and caregivers seemingly not relating with one another).

→ *Medicalization* ("the invocation of a medical diagnosis explaining symptoms without evidence of disease and the application of medical intervention to treat them") is widespread.

→ The patient/doctor relationship is threatened by multiple influences.

→ Many people do not trust doctors.

→ The individual must be responsible for his/her health.

Life is perplexing, arduous, and very stressful. You weren't biologically designed to live it this way, so you're symptomatic. Even if it isn't apparent to you, this is the way it is for everybody. You are not alone.

YOU must understand and accept your responsibility to Regain Balance and FIND HEALTH. It's all about YOU.

THE BIOPSYCHOSOCIAL MODEL

You now know that in a perfect world, the biopsychosocial model would be used by both patients and doctors. You also understand the reality. It is rarely used.

DOCTOR-CENTERED APPROACH

Most doctors were trained to elicit symptoms of disease using a doctor-centered approach. The physician takes charge of the interaction to meet her or his own needs of eliciting symptoms, their details, and other information that will allow diagnosis. Personal concerns are largely ignored and discouraged so that the doctor can focus upon making a diagnosis. The doctor takes the lead from the patient and prevents the expression of most personal information by the patient. This is one of several ways in which the biopsychosocial model is not utilized.

PATIENT-CENTERED INTERVIEWING

But you're in charge. An isolated focus upon the symptoms by both you and your doctor is counterproductive. It is important to express what is most important to you, including personal ideas, concerns, and emotions. Sandeep Jauhar, M.D. is a cardiologist in Long Island, New York and the author of *Intern: A Doctor's Initiation.* In an article published in *The New York Times* on January 6, 2009, "The Instincts to Trust Are Usually the Patient's," he writes that the best instincts in medicine derive from the patients themselves. He says, "Their intuitions about their own health may be denigrated by doctors." His conclusion is that his patients have taught him "they often hold the vital clue."

Regarding your symptoms and health, we recommend that you relay the following to your doctor.

Ideas

"Here's my opinion on what is wrong with me."

"I want you to know what's been going on in my life because it may have something to do with what's wrong with me."

Vanderbilt's Dr. Clifton Meador advised medical students and doctors in training to ask the patient what s/he suspected might be wrong because they often know. Do not hesitate to give your own opinion about your symptoms and health.

Concerns

"I'm concerned about what may be wrong with me."

This can be different than offering your ideas and opinion. You might not believe that you have cancer. Yet you may be worried about the possibility. It is important that your doctor and/or caregiver knows your concerns to reassure you about what you do and do not have wrong.

Emotions

Do not be afraid to express them.

"I'm so upset by these symptoms that I can't sleep and my husband doesn't have any patience with me."

Anxiety/Depression?

Be honest with yourself. In the following section, we will provide you with the tools to explore the possibility that you are suffering with anxiety, depression, or both.

You may need to help your doctor with this. The power must be shared so that you can develop autonomy. This type of relationship with your doctor will help you develop a sense of self-sufficiency and responsibility. When you both recognize the importance of personal, emotional and social concerns that influence your perceptions, understanding, acceptance, and treatment, you stand to benefit.

DO YOU HAVE ANXIETY AND/OR DEPRESSION?

In **PART 1**, you learned about the strong association between depression and medically unexplained symptoms, symptom syndromes, like irritable bowel syndrome and fibromyalgia, and serious diseases, including metabolic syndrome and coronary artery disease. Scientific studies show that even though patients suffering with depression and anxiety usually describe medically unexplained physical symptoms, most will also admit to experiencing psychological/emotional symptoms only if doctors specifically ask them. While sophisticated psychological screening and diagnostic tools are available to doctors, most outside the mental health professions do not use them. The reason they give is that they don't have time.

We think that screening tools for depression and anxiety may be useful to YOU.

Dr. Kurt Kroenke's "S4" Model for Predicting Presence of Depression and Anxiety

→ High physical symptom count (greater than five)
→ Recent stress (yes/no)
→ Low self-rated health of poor or fair on a five-point scale (excellent, very good, good, fair, poor)
→ Self-rated severity of presenting symptom(s) of six or greater on a zero (none) to ten (unbearable) scale
→ The presence of any of these four predictors increases the odds by at least two to threefold that there is an underlying depressive or anxiety disorder. Furthermore, the effect is additive, with the prevalence of a depressive or anxiety disorder being only five percent in patients with no S4 predictor, seventeen percent in those with one predictor, forty-one percent in those with two predictors, seventy percent in those with three predictors, and ninety-four percent in those patients with all four predictors.

Anxiety Screen (GAD-2)

Dr. Kroenke and colleagues have developed a generalized anxiety disorder (GAD-2) screen for anxiety disorders, the most common of which are post-traumatic stress disorder, generalized anxiety disorder, panic disorder, and social anxiety disorder. Two questions are included in the GAD-2 screening tool:

1. "Over the last two weeks, how often have you been bothered by the following problems: feeling nervous, anxious, or on edge?"

2. "Over the last two weeks, how often have you been bothered by the following problem: not being able to stop worrying?"

The total score is based upon responses ranging from "not at all" (0), "several days" (1), "more than half the days" (2), and "nearly every day" (3). A score of 3 or higher suggests presence of a possible anxiety disorder.

Depression Screen (PHQ-2)

Dr. Kroenke and colleagues have also developed a screen for depression based upon two questions (PHQ-2):

1. "Over the past two weeks, have you felt down, depressed, or hopeless?"

2. "Over the past two weeks, have you felt little interest or pleasure in doing things?"

The PHQ-2 inquires about the frequency of depressed mood over the past two weeks with responses and scoring as described for GAD-2, scoring each as "not at all" (0), to "nearly every day" (3). A PHQ-2 score of 3 or higher had a sensitivity of 83 percent and specificity of 92 percent for major depression. The PHQ-2 is available on the Internet (see **Bibliography**).

DO YOU HAVE METABOLIC SYNDROME?

If you do, it is essential that you understand your condition and the self-care behaviors you must apply. Two excellent resources are included in the **Bibliography**: Dr. Arthur Agatston's book, *The South Beach Heart Health Revolution*, and (if you want medical detail), "A Practical "ABCDE" Approach to the Metabolic Syndrome," a medical article in Mayo Clinic Proceedings.

PERSONAL HEALTH RECORD (MEDICAL RECORD)

Two major companies have focused upon the fragmentation, duplication, and lack of portability characterizing the current paper-based medical system. They have developed Internet-based personal health records (PHR). Microsoft launched HealthVault in the fall of 2007, and Google launched Google Health in the spring of 2008. These personal health records provide individuals with secure, user-friendly systems for aggregating all of their health records, data, diagnostic images, laboratory results, and medical histories.

Whether or not you use a PHR, you should have a typed and updated version of your medical history available for all of your doctors and caregivers, which includes:

- *Chief complaint*

  Write out a description of your symptoms including when they began, where they are located, and whether they are getting worse. Include your ideas, concerns, emotions, and opinions regarding the presence of anxiety and/or depression.

- *Past medical history*

- *Past surgical history*

- *Medications with dosage and frequency (everything, including over the counter, "natural," and herbal products)*

- *Allergies, including medications*

- *Social history*

  Include occupation; marital status; tobacco use (type and amount per day on average; and any history of former use); alcohol intake (type and amount per day on average; and any history of former use); and recreational drug use, including previous use.

- *Review of symptoms*

  These are the symptoms not necessarily related to your chief complaint and reason for the visit. For example, if you come to a gastroenterologist because of abdominal pain associated with bowel dysfunction, you may also have other symptoms such as fatigue, problems sleeping, and pain all over your body. These are symptoms that should be familiar to you and be made known to your doctor since they may result in a diagnosis of irritable bowel syndrome and fibromyalgia syndrome.

FAMILY HISTORY

By now, you understand that your health is related to your family history. The following is quoted from the United States Department of Health &

Human Services U. S. Surgeon General's Family History Initiative Internet site:

Health care professionals have known for a long time that common diseases—heart disease, cancer, and diabetes—and rare diseases—like hemophilia, cystic fibrosis, and sickle cell anemia—can run in families. If one generation of a family has high blood pressure, it is common for the next generation to have similarly high blood pressure. Tracing the illnesses suffered by your parents, grandparents, and other blood relatives can help your doctor predict the disorders to which you may be at risk and take action to keep you and your family healthy.

To help focus attention on the importance of family history, the surgeon general, in cooperation with other agencies with the U.S. Department of Health and Human Services, has launched a national public health campaign, called the Surgeon General's Family History Initiative, to encourage all American families to learn more about their family health history.

The Internet site provides a free tool called "My Family Health Portrait," which is a web-enabled program that runs on any computer connected to the web and running an up-to-date version of any major Internet browser. The web-based tool helps users organize family history information and then print it out for presentation to their caregivers. In addition, the tool helps users save their family history information to their own computer and even share family history information with other family members.

MEDICATIONS, INCLUDING ANTIDEPRESSANTS

There are many drugs and treatments available for medically unexplained symptoms, functional somatic syndromes, anxiety, and depression. Our Still Hurting? FIND HEALTH Series™ will address diagnosis and management of these diseases, and you can visit our Internet site:

www.stillhurtingfindhealth.com

These drugs can be either approved by the Food and Drug Administration (FDA) or be approved for other indications but used to treat the functional somatic syndrome off-label. For example, antidepressant drugs are not only used with FDA approval to treat depression, but are also used off-label to treat medically unexplained symptoms, including chronic pain and functional somatic syndromes.

While doctors recommend such off-label use of antidepressants to relieve chronic pain and bodily symptoms, most patients don't understand why they should take an antidepressant for this purpose. Frankly, many are offended. Some refuse to do so.

Attempting to help patients understand, noted gastroenterologist Douglas A. Drossman, M.D. (recall that you learned about him in Chapter 9) offers a patient educational handout entitled *The Use of Antidepressants in the Treatment of Irritable Bowel Syndrome and Other Functional GI Disorders* (Internet site from the University of North Carolina Center for Functional GI & Motility Disorders) referenced in the **Bibliography**. Antidepressants can help reduce bodily symptoms by affecting the four mind/brain systems:

BODY TALK: control of bodily sensitivity, distress, and autonomic reactivity;

STRESS: maintenance and balance of the stress response;

EMOTIONS: mood alteration; and

CONSCIOUSNESS: impact on positive thinking and negative thoughts.

Dr. Kurt Kroenke and colleagues have recently reviewed the use of antidepressants for eleven symptom syndromes: irritable bowel syndrome, chronic back pain, headache, fibromyalgia, chronic fatigue syndrome, tinnitus, menopausal symptoms, chronic facial pain, noncardiac chest pain, interstitial cystitis, and chronic pelvic pain. They conclude, "For some syndromes, the data for or against treatment effectiveness is relatively robust, for many, however, the data, one way or the other is scanty."

The point is that treatment with antidepressants may or may not be helpful for medically unexplained symptoms and symptom syndromes.

Recall that from neuroimaging findings, recent research provides evidence that various mind/brain–based therapies, including hypnotherapy, cognitive behavioral therapy, and placebo, all involve engagement of these same mind/brain systems that are potentially affected by antidepressant drugs. Combination treatment, such as cognitive behavioral therapy in addition to antidepressant drug therapy, may be more beneficial than either alone. If you choose to take antidepressant drugs to help relieve distressing symptoms, you will now have a clearer understanding of what you are doing.

YOU'RE IN CHARGE

In conclusion, you have the ability to become proactive about your health. Learn all the family medical history you can. Keep and consolidate your personal medical information. When you must see a doctor, come prepared with your questions and concerns. If you choose to take medication or you and your doctor determine that you must, know why. By understanding what is behind your symptoms, you begin to see clearly and are much more likely to benefit from treatment. This reinvigorates trust; and restoring the doctor-patient relationship is a task that needs to be shared. After all, it's your health that is at issue.

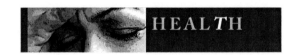

Team with All Care-Givers

Each of us enjoys walking the beach. The sand provides physical resistance while the water soothes the soul. WBS now lives near the beach. TLH's favorite beach is at least a long day's drive away. Living in central Ohio, he has to improvise if he wants to walk by the water. One option is a bike and hiking trail along the Scioto River. Meandering through the downtown and northwest suburbs, the Scioto is one of the few spots for water activities in Columbus. Because it's not a very wide river, fishermen vie with skiers for trolling and slaloming space.

On weekends, the number of boats multiplies, as do the walkers and incontinent geese. North of Griggs Dam, rowing takes over a section of the river as four and eight-person shells compete in high school and college regattas. Walking alongside the watercourse offers a good vantage point to take in the teamwork of the rowers. In many races, each boat has a coxswain, the crewmember responsible for steering and guiding the shell. He or she navigates the course and synchronizes the rhythm and muscle of the rowers. When they are in sync, their cadenced propulsion is impressive. The rowers team their strength and their oar-handling finesse while the coxswain, like a good point guard or music conductor, coordinates movement and flow. Walking on the riverbank and glancing at the finish, you can't help but marvel over the synergy of the lead team.

WHAT TEAM?

You simply don't see many other examples of the precision teamwork it requires to succeed in a crew. We certainly haven't witnessed it in our work. As previously described, medical care suffers from disjointedness and fragmentation. And ministers are often in the dark about who else may be involved professionally in a parishioner's care.

Even though doctors share a common training, they often exhibit a limited ability to coordinate efforts. The more specialists added to the team, the harder it becomes to pull in the same direction regarding a patient's care and treatment. Each specialty pursues its own course of action without benefit of one take-charge coxswain who would navigate and steer the whole crew.

Patients with associated symptoms and symptom syndromes don't know who's calling the shots.

The situation is further exacerbated when caregivers from various disciplines are part of a person's care. There may be little or no awareness of one another, let alone that they are supposed to be teaming up to propel the same boat.

WHAT DIAGNOSIS?

Often, only one person has any idea who all the players are and how disjointed their effort may be. Unfortunately, it's the care-receiver. When you are symptomatic, differently diagnosed, and variously advised, it is YOU.

In Chapter 8, we quote Dr. Paul W. Pruyser, who apprises correctly that any person's symptoms diagnosis depends altogether upon who is doing the diagnosing.

Medical doctors, especially specialists, deduce and diagnose based on their area of expertise. Counselors practice different disciplines and counseling techniques. Dentists talk teeth and gums. Certain practitioners of alternative medicine pinpoint problems, provide homeopathic remedies, or manipulate the spine. Clerics engage matters of the spirit and search the soul. Whether they are cognizant of each other's presence in a care-receiver's life is often nebulous. Who knows the others are there?

WHAT TREATMENT? WHAT CARE?

Moreover, the remedies and treatments they offer will also derive from their area of practice. They may or may not mix well. Prescription medications may interact poorly, thereby compromising each prescriber's approach. If there is no coordination of medications, the patient may be left unknowing or confused.

Counselors' advice may not mesh when several disciplines are involved. Clergy who need to be all things to all people stay in counseling relationships when they are beyond the limits of spiritual expertise and out of their depths. Hopefully, they refer. Psychologists with a bias toward a certain technique may not fully explore matters of the spirit and soul. If both disciplines remain involved in a person's care, the approaches may vary wildly.

Finally, there is the potential for "Who's on first?" confusion if you find yourself hospitalized with multiple symptoms and/or associated syndromes. As various doctors of different persuasions appear and disappear from bed-ridden view, you and those close to you wonder, "Who's in charge?" If you're not sure, and can't even keep their names straight, you are likely better off asking the nurses to steer you true. Be the fragmented care inner-disciplinary or multi-disciplinary, you may think that there is no way to get a handle on coordinating your health care. Believing this to be true, it will remain your premise as long as you do nothing to alter the angle of your point of view.

SEE YOURSELF IN CHARGE

Consider looking at the issue of your health care teamwork not from the perspective of a "can't do anything about it" victim, but from that of the proactive, take-charge agent of your own well-being.

How do you get there from here? Initially, you have three challenges:

1. Begin to see yourself as the connect-the-dots handcrafter of your own health care;

2. Get beyond (UNLEARN) seeing yourself as a health care consumerist; and

3. Re-examine the idea that the experts on body, mind/brain, and soul have such a knowledge advantage over you that you can't talk with them about your health.

Wrestling with these challenges isn't easy. After all, you've been conditioned to receive and consume health care from the experts. However, at the center of your care isn't someone who only has office times to see you.

YOU are at the center of your care! It is your mind/brain, body, and soul at issue. Who engages how and what you feel more than you? You are the key figure. The caregivers are the supporting cast.

Reflect again upon the description of the rowers on the river. Imagine you are the coxswain and your health care providers are the rest of the crew.

The rudder is in your hands. You are directing the rhythms of their work because you are speaking up, even if you need a megaphone to find your voice. To the cadence you dictate, they respond.

Together, you are a team intent on steering a course to regain balance and FIND HEALTH.

Team members include your physician(s), spiritual advisor(s), dentist, and counselors and alternative medicine practitioners, if any. They are aware of one another because you have taken charge, made them aware, and when necessary for your well-being, consented to their interaction. (Note regarding consent: certain personal privacy matters may involve legal issues, including any privilege that exists between professional caregivers and you. When questions arise on the sharing of personal information, consult an attorney.) They take their cues from you.

Can you imagine it? You can do more than imagine; you can build your team. Keeping in mind the three initial challenges we have already outlined, you can foster team building among all your caregivers by:

→ investing yourself in learning how they think (especially doctors, as discussed in the previous section);
→ compiling your health history and sharing it because it's what you don't know or they don't know that can hurt you;
→ making them aware of medical, spiritual, emotional, and personal/ social issues in your life, which affect their respective disciplines and may necessitate their collaboration; and
→ continuing to learn how your symptoms and associated syndromes overlap and require a collaborative, synergistic effort to deal with them.

While all of these points are important parts of team building, the last one in particular may save your life. We close this section by posing an example of a symptoms linkage you may not have given much thought to or even are aware of. From *Crest* toothpaste ads and trips to the dentist, you know your oral hygiene is very important. You know the drill of brushing and flossing regularly. But do you know that there is a link between periodontal disease and heart disease? People with gum disease are twice as likely to have coronary artery disease. If your gums are infected, your entire body suffers from the inflammation triggered by the immune response. According to an article published in the December 2007 issue of *The Journal of Periodontology*, the authors conclude that long-term bacterial exposure from gum disease accounts for increased cardiac risk. The common denominator is the inflammation. The linkage between gum and heart disease is strong.

Think about it. Would you normally talk to your dentist about your heart?

Perhaps you will because now you know how symptoms can overlap and otherwise be tied to one another.

Thus, you begin to realize how necessary it is for you to take charge of your health. One way you do that is by teaming with all your caregivers to regain balance and FIND HEALTH.

This is a task for which you are now better suited because you don't see yourself as alone in this anymore.

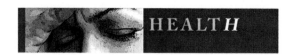

Help Others Help Themselves

When you are symptomatic, you likely have occasions in which someone offers an opinion on how to fix the problem. Perhaps it's a long-time friend. He or she's well meaning, but may not be too strong on listening skills. As you haltingly describe the pain you're feeling, your friend breaks in to prescribe a solution. The prescription is based less on what you have been saying than on what this person filters through his or her own experience. In a way, he or she is trying to relate to you by comparing stories, but the relating falls short. Listening is hard work. It hurts. In your friend's preoccupation with thinking about how to respond, he or she stops listening and grasps for resolution. Your story becomes your friend's. The pain remains. Maybe you just won't go there the next time you talk. When you think about it, many conversations go just like the one with the friend. People want to resolve your problem instead of listening and encouraging you to sort through whatever's behind your symptoms. This happens continuously; and for different reasons, you find it to be the case when you seek professional consultation as well.

IN DOCTORS' OFFICES, YOU SENSE IMPATIENCE

Part of it you sense from the physicians who practice on the clock. Part of it is yours as you grapple with being concise. You find yourself boxed into a medical repair shop cubicle in which the conversation is short and the quick fix is the remedy of time-constrained choice. There's simply no time for much else.

But even when there is time for listening and exploration, few take it. You feel the press of black and white yearnings in a gray world. Few have the patience and maturity to live with unsettling complexity. Fewer appear to have the capacity to listen well. You sense it even among those closest to you. They mean well. They care for you. They can't bear seeing you in pain. They want to resolve the issue—fix the problem. But they can't. It is your health at issue, not theirs.

While you know by reading this book that you are ultimately the one responsible for regaining your balance, you also know from experience that isolation and aloneness are not conducive to finding health. Yes, you need time for solitude and reflection. You also need to avoid conversations with fixers. However, becoming reclusive, with only your symptoms for company, is not a strategy for success. Alone and left to your own devices, you are susceptible to denial, depression, and delusion. Whether you think of yourself as a victim or the captain of your soul, you cannot find health in a vacuum. Instead, you need to be part of a community in which you can accept empathetic care from others and help others help themselves.

Paradoxically, the dual dynamics of receiving and giving are beneficial to your own well-being. One without the other does not suffice. If all you do is give yourself away to others, you find yourself fatigued and spent. You may also become incapable of any self-realization apart from defining yourself by your ability to meet others' needs and expectations. There is simply no YOU left because you have given yourself away. On the other hand, if you only take in and do not give and get outside yourself, you may end up with a sense of self completely dependent upon the enabling it takes to prop it up. Sorely dependant on the enabling of others, you find yourself with no core, will, or resolve of your own.

Finding the capacity to both give and receive fleshes out a YOU who fears neither solitude nor social life. There is emerging balance. As you find yourself accepting real help (not cheap advice and fix-it remedies), you become better acclimated to the listening skills and empathy it takes to deliver care and make it real. You absorb it, make it your model, and emerge as a growing, empathetic good listener. You are able to get outside yourself and give care, even as you are able to accept the care and wise counsel of others.

By using your own personal experiences of what has been helpful and what has not, you build a foundation for helping others help themselves. This has the double benefit of feeding and reinforcing both your own self-care and that of others. You are listening to and empathizing with them and that is a sign of respect. You offer no cheap advice. You have no need to fix them or resolve their problems. Instead, you respect them to do for themselves what you are doing for yourself by taking charge of your own health.

Consider how much the world around you needs you to do just that.

In 2007, representatives of twenty-nine nations gathered in Singapore to attend a conference on "Medically Unexplained Symptoms in Family Life." Topics included formulation of a broadly acceptable definition of MUS; creation of better, earlier MUS recognition strategies; and patient self-management and empowerment. For all the wisdom and experience of those gathered, they concluded that more research was necessary to determine why medical consultations with MUS patients are so unsatisfactory and problematic. They agreed to research what you and millions of people with MUS already know!

WHEN IT COMES TO DIAGNOSING AND DISCUSSING MEDICALLY UNEXPLAINED SYMPTOMS, MEDICINE DOESN'T HAVE IT TOGETHER

Its approach is linear and fragmented. It sees patients like you in fragmented perspective. It settles for trying to fix medically unexplained symptoms with a label, a prescription, and a referral. Seeing that, you see the truth.

YOU understand you can't rely on care-giving fixers, whatever their stripe.

Answer churches don't allow for your doubts and questions. Doctors don't have time to listen. Other caregivers seem to fixate on just a part of you.

Your health is up to you.

Since you know this is the case, you are in position to respectfully share with others what you have found for yourself. You know others who hurt. You can sense younger generations beginning to be symptomatic. You've seen the signs of stress in the children or grandchildren in your family or in the neighborhood kids. You're right about what you sense in them. It is critically important to share knowledge about being symptomatic with those who are in the early stages of their lives. Your empathy may help encourage them to regain their balance and find health.

We conclude with an example of why this is necessary. Each year, Bexley High School in Columbus, Ohio invites an alumnus to participate in the Dr. Judah Folkman Scientist-in-Residence Program. For a week, WBS served as a resident medical scientist, interacting with students and faculty. In preparation, WBS asked one of the principals, Earl Focht, the following question:

"Are high school students stressed out and symptomatic?"

His answer,

"Very."

You are not surprised by the answer. Looking behind your symptoms, you've discovered that sometimes you start hurting when you are young and vulnerable. Without guidance and understanding, the pain doesn't go away. Stress builds. Kids become symptomatic. They need role models who remember, understand, empathize, and teach them well. One of them could be you. You think of the younger people around you and what the future holds if they remain over-stressed and out of balance. As you ponder how to regain balance, you remember the acronym FIND HEALTH and, reaching back, pull from memory that last H.

Help Others Help Themselves

You look for ways to put it into practice.

Perhaps you recommend our book.

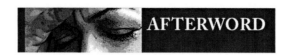

AFTERWORD

We have written **PART 4** neither as a ten-step program nor as a recipe for self-help. From our experience, we don't believe that everybody can Regain Balance and FIND HEALTH by following each other in lock step.

Life is a messy learning process. People vary in their hurt. What lies behind your symptoms is personal to you.

Therefore, we hope you will find an array of points of entry in seeking to regain your balance. It is not necessary to approach the **PART 4** material systematically. In applying the sections on finding your muse, imagining your own wellness, and nurturing yourself, we encourage your freedom and creativity. You may find some concepts more accessible than others. Don't worry if that happens. These areas are meant to trigger your individuality. It is up to you.

However, the sections on dining well, holding your weight down, exercising, adding vitamins and supplements, learning, teaming, and helping others have universal application. Each of us needs to find ways to include them in a personal health regimen. If you find yourself struggling with a given topic, that's okay. Keep at it and don't give up on all the others just because one proves difficult.

Remember, you are not alone in your symptoms.

We are with you on this and hope that you will continue to interact with us by visiting our website regularly and joining the Still Hurting? FIND HEALTH! ™ community:

stillhurtingfindhealth.com

About the Authors

L ifelong friends, the authors are two caregivers from diverse healing traditions, each of whom has an extensive professional background. Both doctors and ministers have the humbling privilege of accessing the heart and soul of the human condition. They encounter pain, hurt, and *dis-ease* as multidimensional dysfunction and often puzzling, symptomatic imbalance. The authors' complementary experience inspired them personally and professionally to come together and offer this book after over six years of collaboration.

William B. Salt II, M.D.

William B. Salt II, M.D. is board-certified in both internal medicine and gastroenterology. He received his M.D. degree from The Ohio State University in Columbus, Ohio, in 1972, where he holds an appointment as Clinical Assistant Professor in Medicine. He trained for five additional years in internal medicine and gastroenterology at Vanderbilt University Hospitals in Nashville, Tennessee, where he also served as a Chief Resident in Medicine. He returned home to Columbus, Ohio and practiced gastroenterology 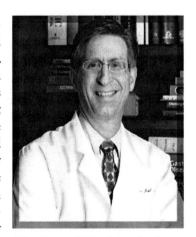 for 33 years. Dr. Salt's primary hospital was Mt. Carmel Health, which is a teaching hospital and affiliate of The Ohio State University.

His awards and honors include:
- → Mount Carmel 2009 Physician of the Year
- → Dr. Judah Folkman Scientist in Residence at his alma mater, Bexley High School in Columbus, Ohio in 2003

→ Distinguished Educator of the Year 2000 by The Ohio State University
→ Mount Carmel Family Practice Residency Teacher of the Year, 1995–1996 (first nonfamily practice physician recipient)
→ Mount Carmel Teacher of the Year in Medicine, 1978–1979
→ Regularly included in Best Doctors in America®

Dr. Salt is the author of the first edition and coauthor of the revised edition of *Irritable Bowel Syndrome and the MindBodySpirit Connection* and *Fibromyalgia and the MindBodySpirit Connection*. He has written numerous medical journal articles and several chapters in books for physicians and health care professionals.

Thomas L. Hudson, M.Div., J.D.

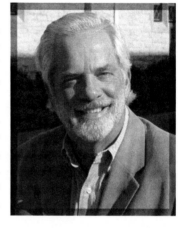

Reverend Thomas L. Hudson is a 1973 honors graduate of Trinity Lutheran Seminary in Columbus, Ohio. He also holds a J.D. degree from Capital University Law School where he graduated "magna cum laude."

With a passion for both the law and ministry, he has interacted with thousands of needful people. For twenty-five years, he served churches across the spectrum of geography, culture, and ethnicity. He began his ministry in Clovis, New Mexico. Trained there as a volunteer police chaplain, he was on call twenty-four hours a day. The 3:00 a.m. emergency phone calls shaped his ministry and honed his empathy for those who were broken and lived on the edge.

He later served in New Orleans and Columbus, his home town. Always community focused, he has been a crisis intervention counselor, guest lecturer, and board chair for both the Franklin County Child Abuse and Child Neglect Advisory Board and Lutheran Social Services of Central Ohio, the second largest non-profit agency in the Columbus area.

Our Story

Over the course of our careers, we often contemplated and discussed working together. As we finished the book that had preoccupied us for six years, we looked at one another in wonder as we reflected upon the source of its inspiration. In gratitude, we want to share our story on how and why we came to write it.

Lifelong friends, we are two caregivers from divergent professions. Over the years, we have had many conversations in which we pondered our collective recognition of the pain evidenced in stories shared by our patients, parishioners, and friends—and in our own shared health experiences. These histories were full of multiple medically unexplained symptoms expressed as pain, discomfort, fatigue, insomnia, depression, anxiety, obsessions, repressions, and compulsions. Many were struggling with being overweight and some with related complications, such as metabolic syndrome. Some had potentially harmful behaviors and habits. Most had seen more than one professional.

Questions and expectations abounded. "What's causing my pain and symptoms?" "Fix me; I'm broken." Ironically, we had to become symptomatic ourselves to begin asking the right questions to discover the right answers. We came to understand that *dis-ease* was dysfunction embodied as symptoms involving both the body and mind/brain. The problem could be understood only from a viewpoint that honors the complex interrelationships of science, medicine, psychology, spirituality, and religion. Realizing that the time to share what we'd learned individually and collaboratively had finally come, we wrote this book. And we'll continue our exploration as long as the spirit moves us and we are able.

We come from medicine and the ministry, although TLH remarkably managed to earn a law degree in his "spare time" (graduating from law school *magnum cum laude*). He taught law for several years while serving full-time in parish ministry. Having served five churches, he is a wise teacher and counselor.

WBS intended to become a primary care physician, having been inspired by his doctor, Howard "Bud" Mitchell, until he concluded that there was too much to know. He decided to specialize as an internist and ultimately become a subspecialist. Gastroenterology is a technical field, much of which involves the performance of endoscopic procedures. But the primary care doctor at heart became increasingly distressed because the causes of abdominal pain and gastrointestinal symptoms often didn't show up on tests. He thought,

Well, then, all the more important to spend time understanding the patient's story and help him or her discover what's behind the symptoms.

Thereafter, he wrote three books for patients, intending to help them while relieving some of his own discomfiture. While beginning to write this book, he knew there was an essential missing dimension, which he believed in strongly but did not have the education, experience, talent, and skill to articulate. He knew where to go for help and invited his coauthor to join the endeavor.

Doctors and ministers have the great privilege of accessing the heart and soul of the human condition. As we shared stories *of dis-ease* over the years, we came to know that the epidemic of symptoms involves each of us in multidimensional ways. Body, mind, and soul are all linked and impacted. Those suffering consult with a variety of caregivers in multiple disciplines. But their care is fragmented. The focus is upon expedient treatment rather than self-discovery of the healing power within. While the two of us have our differences—politics for one—we share certain core beliefs that nourish and inspire us. These include faith in God, recognition of grace, and gratitude for the power of love. We believe in wholeness and integration rather than separateness and fragmentation.

Scientist, philosopher, and Jesuit priest Pierre Teilhard de Chardin includes two core ideas in *Phenomenon of Man*. For us, particularly as caregivers, they are much more than ideas. On *Science and Spirituality*, he writes, "They are both relevant to the whole of human existence. The religiously minded can no longer turn their backs upon the natural world. Nor can the materialistic-minded deny importance to spiritual experiences and religious feelings." On *Wholeness and Convergence*, he says that our field of vision should extend to the whole and "like the meridians as they approach the poles, science, philosophy, and religion are bound to converge as they draw nearer to the whole." From such convergence will emerge "the organic whole in which no element can any longer be separated from those surrounding it."

Dis-ease is multidimensional dysfunction and imbalance manifested as symptoms. This realization has inspired us personally and professionally to come together and offer this book. By understanding symptoms through the complexity of the whole perspective of convergent science, philosophy, and spirituality/religion, every one of us can be optimistic about the opportunities for finding health.

William B. Salt II, M.D.
Sanibel, Florida

Thomas L. Hudson, M.Div., J.D.
Columbus, Ohio

March 15, 2011

Introduction

Carmichael M. "Healthy at Any Age." *Newsweek.* June 28 & July 5, 2010.

PubMed (PubMed is a service of the U.S. National Library of Medicine). Available at: www.pubmed.gov. Accessed 2 April, 2011.

Eliot TS. *The Rock.* London: Faber & Faber, 1934.

Radner G. *It's Always Something: Twentieth Anniversary Edition.* New York: Simon & Schuster, 2009.

Peck MS. *The Road Less Traveled, 25th Anniversary Edition (A New Psychology of Love, Traditional Values, and Spiritual Growth).* New York: Touchstone, 2003.

Lewis CS. *The Problem of Pain.* New York: HarperOne, 2001.

Menninger K, Mayman M, Pruyser P. *The Vital Balance: The Life Process in Mental Health and Illness.* New York: Viking, 1963.

Kuhn TS. *The Structure of Scientific Revolutions (Third Edition).* Chicago: University of Chicago Press, 1996 (first published in 1962).

Sagan C, Druyan A. *The Demon-Haunted World: Science as a Candle in the Dark.* New York: Random House, 1996.

PART 1
THE EPIDEMIC OF SYMPTOMS

Chapter 1
YOU are Symptomatic

Menninger K, Mayman M, Pruyser P. *The Vital Balance: The Life Process in Mental Health and Illness.* New York: Viking, 1963.

Merikangas KR, Ames M, Cui L, Stang PE, Ustun TB, Von Korff M, Kessler RC. "The impact of comorbidity of mental and physical conditions on role disability in the US adult household population." *Arch Gen Psychiatry.* 2007 Oct; 64(10):1180-8.

Verbrugge LM, Ascione FJ. "Exploring the iceberg. Common symptoms and how people care for them." *Med Care.* 1987 Jun; 25(6):539-69.

Kroenke K. "Unburdening the difficult clinical encounter." *Arch Intern Med.* 2009; 169(4):333-4.

An PG, Rabatin JS, Manwell LB, Linzer M, Brown RL, Schwartz MD; MEMO Investigators. "Burden of difficult encounters in primary care: data from the minimizing error, maximizing outcomes study." *Arch Intern Med.* 2009 Feb 23; 169(4):410-4.

Barsky AJ, Borus JF. "Somatization and medicalization in the era of managed care." *JAMA.* 1995 Dec 27; 274(24):1931-4.

Conrad P. *The Medicalization of Society: On the Transformation of Human Conditions into Treatable Disorders.* Baltimore: The Johns Hopkins University Press, 2007.

Chapter 2
We (the Authors) Are Symptomatic Too

The Papers of Thomas Jefferson, Vol 11. ed. Julian P. Boyd. Princeton, NJ: Princeton University Press, 1955, p. 558.

Chapter 3
There's a Symptom Epidemic, and We're All In It

Komaroff A. "Symptoms: in the head or in the brain?" *Ann Intern Med.* 2001 May 1; 134(9 [Part 1]):783-5.

"Investigating symptoms: frontiers in primary care research-perspectives from the seventh Regenstrief conference." *Ann Intern Med.* 2001 May 1; 134(9 [Part 2]):801-930.

Sarno J. *The MindBody Prescription: Healing the Body, Healing the Pain.* New York: Grand Central Publishing (formerly Warner Books), 1998.

Sarno J. *The Divided Mind: The Epidemic of MindBody Disorders.* New York: Harper Paperbacks, 2007.

Hammond EC. "Some preliminary findings on physical complaints from a prospective study of 1,064,004 men and women." *Am J Public Health Nations Health.* 1964 Jan; 54:11-23.

Sandler RS, Stewart WF, Liberman JN, Ricci JA, Zorich NL. "Abdominal pain, bloating, and diarrhea in the United States: prevalence and Impact." *Dig Dis Sci.* 2000 Jun; 45(6):1166-71.

Lipsitz JD, Masia-Warner C, Apfel H, Marans Z, Hellstern B, Forand N,

Levenbraun Y, Fyer AJ. "Anxiety and depressive symptoms and anxiety sensitivity in youngsters with noncardiac chest pain and benign heart murmurs." *J Pediatr Psychol.* 2004 Dec; 29(8):607-12.

Lipsitz JD, Masia C, Apfel H, Marans Z, Gur M, Dent H, Fyer AJ. "Noncardiac chest pain and psychopathology in children and adolescents." *J Psychosom Res.* 2005 Sep; 59(3):185-8.

Lateef TM, Merikangas KR, He J, Kalaydjian A, Khoromi S, Knight E, Nelson KB. "Headache in a national sample of American children: prevalence and comorbidity." *J Child Neurol.* 2009 May; 24(5):536-43.

Schwille IJ, Giel KE, Ellert U, Zipfel S, Enck P. "A community-based survey of abdominal pain prevalence, characteristics, and health care use among children." *Clin Gastroenterol Hepatol.* 2009 Oct; 7(10):1062-8. Epub 2009 Aug 9.

Rask CU, Olsen EM, Elberling H, Christensen MF, Ornbøl E, Fink P, Thomsen PH,

Skovgaard AM. "Functional somatic symptoms and associated impairment in 5-7-year-old children: the Copenhagen Child Cohort 2000." *Eur J Epidemiol.* 2009; 24(10):625-34. Epub 2009 Jul 26.

Ihlebaek C, Eriksen HR, Ursin H. "Prevalence of subjective health complaints (SHC) in Norway." *Scandinavian J. of Public Health.* 2002; 30(1)20-9.

Sayar K. "Medically unexplained symptoms." *Turk Psikiyatri Derg.* 2002; 13(3):222-31.

Güleç H, Sayar K, Ozkorumak E. "Somatic symptoms of depression." *Turk Psikiyatri Derg.* 2005 Summer; 16(2):90-6.

Eriksen HR, Hellesnes B, Staff P, Ursin H. "Are subjective health complaints a result of modern civilization?" *Int J Behav Med.* 2004; 11(2):122-5.

Reading A. "Illness and disease." *Med Clin N Am.* 1977; 61(4):703-710.

Smith RC, Dwamena FC. "Classification and diagnosis of patients with medically unexplained symptoms." *J Gen Intern Med.* 2007; 22(5):685-91.

Becker E. *The Denial of Death.* New York: Free Press (Simon & Schuster), 1973.

Clauw DJ, Katz P. "The overlap between fibromyalgia and inflammatory rheumatic disease: when and why does it occur?" J Clin Rheumatol. 1995;1:335-342.

Bayless TM, Harris ML. "Inflammatory bowel disease and irritable bowel syndrome." Med Clin North Am. 1990;74:21-28.

Thomas L. *Lives of a Cell: Notes of a Biology Watcher*. New York: Viking Press, 1974.

Chapter 4
Symptoms Lead Us to Doctors and Caregivers

Kroenke K. "The interface between physical and psychological symptoms." *Primary Care Companion. J Clin Psychiatry*. 2003; 5 (suppl 7).

Kroenke K, Rosmalen JG. "Symptoms, syndromes, and the value of psychiatric diagnostics in patients who have functional somatic disorders." *Med Clin N Am*. 2006; 90:603-626.

Shorter F. *Doctors and Their Patients: A Social History*. New Brunswick – U.S.A. and London: Transaction Publishers, 1991.

Barsky AJ, Borus JF. "Somatization and medicalization in the era of managed care." *JAMA*. 1995 Dec 27; 274(24):1931-4.

Kroenke K, Mangelsdorff AD. "Common symptoms in ambulatory care: incidence, evaluation, therapy, and outcome." *American Journal of Medicine*. 1989; 86(3):262-6.

Chapter 5
We Receive a Syndrome Diagnosis

Groopman J. "Hurting all over." In *The New Yorker*. November 13, 2000.

Merriam Webster Online. Available at: www.m-w.com. Accessed 2 April, 2011.

Kroenke K. "Somatic symptoms and depression: a double hurt." *Prim Care Companion J Clin Psychiatry*. 2005; 7:148-149.

Barsky AJ, Borus JF. "Functional somatic syndromes." *Ann Intern Med*. 1999; 130:910-21.

Wessely S, Nimnuan C, Sharpe M. "Functional somatic syndromes: one or many?" *The Lancet*. 1999 Sep 11; 354(9182):936-9.

Diagnostic and Statistical Manual of Mental Disorders. Fourth Edition, Text Revision (DSM-IV-TR). Arlington, VA: American Psychiatric Publishing, Inc., 2000.

Mayes R, Horwitz AV. "DSM-III and the revolution in the classification of mental illness." *J Hist Behav Sci*. 2005; 41(3):249-67.

Katon W, Sullivan M, Walker E. "Medical symptoms without identified pathology: relationship to psychiatric disorders, childhood and adult trauma, and personality traits." *Ann Intern Med*. 2001 May 1; 134(9 [Part 2]):917-25.

Aaron LA, Buchwald D. "A review of the evidence for overlap among unexplained clinical conditions." *Ann Intern Med.* 2001 May 1; 134(9 [Part 2]):868-881.

Schur EA, Afari N, Furberg H, Olarte M, Goldberg J, Sullivan PF, Buchwald D. "Feeling bad in more ways than one: comorbidity patterns of medically unexplained and psychiatric conditions." *J Gen Intern Med.* 2007 Jun; 22(6):818-21.

Horwitz A, Wakefield J. *The Loss of Sadness: How Psychiatry Transformed Normal Sorrow into Depressive Disorder.* New York: Oxford University Press, 2007.

Merikangas KR, Ames M, Cui L, Stang PE, Ustun TB, Von Korff M, Kessler RC. "The impact of comorbidity of mental and physical conditions on role disability in the US adult household population." *Arch Gen Psychiatry.* 2007 Oct; 64(10):1180-8.

Kisely S, Simon G. "An international study comparing the effect of medically explained and unexplained somatic symptoms on psychosocial outcome." *J Psychosom Res.* 2006 Feb; 60(2):125-30.

Chapter 6
The Diagnosis of Depression Describes a Double Hurt

Ovid: *Tristia. Ex Ponto.* (Loeb Classical Library, No. 151).

Kroenke K, Bair MJ, Damush TM, Wu J, Hoke S, Sutherland J, Tu W. "Optimized antidepressant therapy and pain self-management in primary care patients with depression and musculoskeletal pain: a randomized controlled trial." *JAMA.* 2009 May 27; 301(20):2099-110.

Olfson M, Marcus SC." National patterns in antidepressant medication treatment." *Arch Gen Psychiatry.* 2009; 66(8):848-856.

Benson H. *Timeless Healing: The Power and Biology of Belief.* New York: Scribner, 1996.

Taylor S. *Health Psychology (6th edition).* New York: The McGraw-Hill Companies, 2005.

National Institute of Mental Health. Available at: http://www.nimh.nih.gov/index.shtml. Accessed 2 April, 2011.

World Health Organization: Depression. Available at: http://www.who.int/mental_health/management/depression/definition/en/. Accessed 2 April, 2011.

Stewart WF, Ricci JA, Chee E, Morganstein D, Lipton R. "Lost productive time and cost due to common pain conditions in the US workforce." *JAMA.* 2003 Nov 12; 290(18):2443-54.

Gans RO. "The metabolic syndrome, depression, and cardiovascular disease: interrelated conditions that share pathophysiologic mechanisms." *Med Clin North Am.* 2006 Jul; 90:573-91.

Strine TW, Mokdad AH, Dube SR, Balluz LS, Gonzalez O, Berry JT, Manderscheid R, Kroenke K. "The association of depression and anxiety with obesity and unhealthy behaviors among community-dwelling US adults." *Gen Hosp Psychiatry.* 2008 Mar-Apr; 30(2):127-37.

Escobar JI, Interian A, Díaz-Martínez A, Gara M. "Idiopathic physical symptoms: a common manifestation of psychiatric disorders in primary care." *CNS Spectr.* 2006 Mar; 11(3):201-10.

Diagnostic and Statistical Manual of Mental Disorders. Fourth Edition, Text Revision (DSM-IV-TR). Arlington, VA: American Psychiatric Publishing, Inc., 2000.

Henningsen P, Zimmermann T, Sattel H. "Medically unexplained physical symptoms, anxiety, and depression: a meta-analytic review." *Psychosom Med.* 2003 Jul-Aug; 65(4):528-33.

Tylee A, Gandhi P. "The importance of somatic symptoms in depression in primary care." *Prim Care Companion J Clin Psychiatry.* 2005; 7:167-176.

Kroenke K, Rosmalen JG. "Symptoms, syndromes, and the value of psychiatric diagnostics in patients who have functional somatic disorders." *Med Clin North Am.* 2006; 90:603-626.

Whooley MA, Avins AL, Miranda J, Browner WS. "Case-finding instruments for depression: two questions are as good as many." *J Gen Intern Med.* 1997; 12:439-4Kroenke K. "Unburdening the difficult clinical encounter." *Arch Intern Med.* 2009; 169(4):333-4.

Barber C. *Comfortably Numb: How Psychiatry is Medicating a Nation.* New York: Pantheon, 2008.

Bair MJ, Robinson RL, Katon W, Kroenke K. "Depression and pain comorbidity: a literature review." *Arch Intern Med.* 2003 Nov 10; 163(20):2433-45.

Chapter 7
But It's Really a Triple Hurt for Most of Us

Plato. *The Dialogues of Plato, Vol. 1.* Tr. by B. Jowett. London: Oxford University Press, 1892.

Moore T. *Care of the Soul: A Guide for Cultivating Depth and Sacredness in Everyday Life*. New York: HarperCollins Publishers, 1992.

Williams N, Wilkinson C, Stott N, Menkes DB. "Functional illness in primary care: dysfunction versus disease." *BMC Fam Pract*. 2008 May 15; 9:30.

Arizona Center for Integrative Medicine. Available at: http://integrativemedicine.arizona.edu/. Accessed 2 April, 2011.

Duke Integrative Medicine. Available at: http://www.dukeintegrativemedicine.org/. Accessed 2 April, 2011.

Chapter 8
The Diagnosis Doesn't Determine YOUR Health; YOU Do

Baum LF. *The Wonderful Wizard of Oz*. Chicago: George M. Hill Company, 1900.

Pruyser P. *The Minister as Diagnostician: Personal Problems in Pastoral Perspective*. Philadelphia: Westminster John Knox Press, 1976.

Dacher E. *Intentional Healing: A Guide to the Mind-Body Healing System*. New York: Marlowe & Co, 1996.

PART 2
THE BALANCED SELF

Chapter 9
The Complexity of YOUR Life and YOUR Health

Mayer EA. "The challenge of studying the biology of complex, symptom-based GI disorders." *Gastroenterology* 2008; 134:1826-1827.

Meador CK. *Symptoms of Unknown Origin: A Medical Odyssey*. Nashville: Vanderbilt University Press, 2005.

Aristotle. *Aristotle's Metaphysics*. Tr. By J. Sachs. Santa Fe: Green Lion Press, 1999, 2002.

Sarafino E. *Health Psychology: Biopsychosocial Interactions, 5th edition*. New York: Wiley, 2005.

Engel GL. "The need for a new medical model: a challenge for biomedicine." *Science*. 1977; 196(4286):129-36.

Drossman DA. University of North Carolina Center for Functional GI & Motility Disorders. Available at: http://www.med.unc.edu/ibs. Accessed 2 April, 2011.

Cannon WB. *Wisdom of the Body*. New York: W. W. Norton, 1932.

Sterling P, Eyer J. "Allostasis: a new paradigm to explain arousal pathology." In: Fisher S, Reason J, eds. *Handbook of Life Stress, Cognition and Health*. New York: John Wiley, 1988, pages 629-49.

McEwen BS. *The End of Stress As We Know It*. Washington, D. C.: National Academies Press, 2002.

Glass L, Mackey MC. *From Clocks to Chaos, the Rhythms of Life*. Princeton, NJ: Princeton University Press, 1988.

Goldberger AL. "Non-linear dynamics for clinicians: chaos theory, fractals, and complexity at the bedside." *The Lancet*. 1996; 347:1312-4.

Higgins JP. "Nonlinear systems in medicine." *Yale J Biol Med*. 2002 Sep-Dec; 75(5-6):247-60.

Holden LM. "Complex adaptive systems: concept analysis." *J Advanced Nursing*. 2005; 52(6):651-657.

Brown CA. "The role of paradoxical beliefs in chronic pain: a complex adaptive systems perspective." *Nordic College of Caring Science*. 2007; 21(2):207-213.

Resnicow K, Page SE. "Embracing chaos and complexity: a quantum change for public health." *Am J Public Health*. 2008 Aug; 98(8):1382-9. Epub 2008 Jun 12.

Coyle FJ. "'It just doesn't seem to fit.' Environmental illness, corporeal chaos and the body as a complex system." *J Eval Clin Pract*. 2009 Aug; 15(4):770-5.

Rickles D, Hawe P, Shiell A. "A simple guide to chaos and complexity." *J Epidemiol Community Health*. 2007 Nov; 61(11):933-7.

Center for the Study of Biological Complexity, Virginia Commonwealth University. Available at: http://www.vcu.edu/csbc/. Accessed 2 April, 2011.

Chapter 10
How YOU Emerge: Balance and YOUR Internal Environment

Benson H. *Timeless Healing: The Power and Biology of Belief*. New York: Scribner, 1996.

Blakeslee S, Blakeslee M. *The Body Has a Mind of Its Own: How Body Maps in Your Brain Help You Do (Almost) Everything Better*. New York: Random House, 2007.

Proverbs 23:7. *The New American Standard Bible.* La Habra, California: The Lockman Foundation, 1995.

Pert CB. *Molecules of Emotion: Why You Feel the Way You Feel.* New York: Scribner, 1997.

Lane RD, Waldstein SR, Chesney MA, Jennings JR, Lovallo WR, Kozel PJ, Rose RM, Drossman DA, Schneiderman N, Thayer JF, Cameron OG. "The rebirth of neuroscience in psychosomatic medicine, Part I: historical context, methods, and relevant basic science." *Psychosom Med.* 2009 Feb; 71(2):117-34. Epub 2009 Feb 5.

Lane RD, Waldstein SR, Critchley HD, Derbyshire SW, Drossman DA, Wager TD, Schneiderman N, Chesney MA, Jennings JR, Lovallo WR, Rose RM, Thayer JF, Cameron OG. "The rebirth of neuroscience in psychosomatic medicine, Part II: clinical applications and implications for research." *Psychosom Med.* 2009 Feb; 71(2):135-51. Epub 2009 Feb 5.

Mayer EA, Naliboff BD, Craig AD. "Neuroimaging of the brain-gut axis: from basic understanding to treatment of functional GI disorders." *Gastroenterology.* 2006 Dec; 131(6):1925-42.

Craig AD. "Interoception: the sense of the physiological condition of the body." *Curr Opin Neurobiol.* 2003 Aug; 13(4):500-5.

Damasio A. *Descartes' Error: Emotion, Reason, and the Human Brain.* New York: Penguin Group, 2005.

Damasio A. *The Feeling of What Happens: Body and Emotion in the Making of Consciousness.* New York: Houghton Mifflin Harcourt, 2000.

Damasio A. *Looking for Spinoza: Joy, Sorrow, and the Feeling Brain.* New York: Houghton Mifflin Harcourt, 2003.

Craig AD. "A new view of pain as a homeostatic emotion." *Trends Neurosci.* 2003 Jun; 26(6):303-7.

Craig AD. "How do you feel — now? The anterior insula and human awareness." *Nat Rev Neurosci.* 2009 Jan; 10(1):59-70.

Lewis CS. *The Problem of Pain.* New York: HarperOne, 2001.

Lewis CS. *A Grief Observed.* New York: HarperOne, 2001.

Chapter 11
How YOU Emerge: Balance, Heredity, and YOUR External Environment

Hippocrates, *Treatise on Air, Water, and Places.*

Einstein A. as quoted by W. Isaacson in *Einstein: His Life and Universe.* New York: Simon & Schuster, 2007. p.364.

Blakeslee S, Blakeslee M. *The Body Has a Mind of Its Own: How Body Maps in Your Brain Help You Do (Almost) Everything Better*. New York: Random House, 2007.

National Institute of Environmental Health Sciences (NIEHS) – National Institutes of Health/News & Events/2007/04 Sep 2007: Genes, Environment, Health. Available at: http://www.niehs.nih.gov/news/releases/2007/. Accessed 2 April, 2011.

National Institute of Environmental Health Sciences (NIEHS) – National Institutes of Health/Health & Education/Environmental Health Topics/ Environmental Science Basics/Gene-Environment Interaction. Available at: http://www.niehs.nih.gov/health/topics/science/gene-env/index.cfm. Accessed 2 April, 2011.

Paris J. *Nature and Nurture in Psychiatry: A Predisposition – Stress Model of Mental Disorders*. Arlington, VA: American Psychiatric Publishing, Inc., 1999.

Mayer EA. "The challenge of studying the biology of complex, symptom-based GI disorders." *Gastroenterology* 2008; 134:1826-1827.

Guteri F. "Life's complexities." *Newsweek*. July 13, 2009.

Kandel E. "A biology of mental disorder." Newsweek. July 13, 2009.

Dingfelder SF. "The hunt for endophenotypes." *Monitor on Psychology*. 2006; 37:20.

Hasler G, Fromm S, Carlson PJ, Luckenbaugh DA, Waldeck T, Geraci M, Roiser JP, Neumeister A, Meyers N, Charney DS, Drevets WC. "Neural response to catecholamine depletion in unmedicated subjects with major depressive disorder in remission and healthy subjects." *Arch Gen Psychiatry*. 2008 May; 65(5):521-31.

Buskila D, Sarzi-Puttini P. "Biology and therapy of fibromyalgia. Genetic aspects of fibromyalgia syndrome." *Arthritis Res Ther*. 2006; 8(5):218.

Buskila D, Sarzi-Puttini P, Ablin JN. "The genetics of fibromyalgia syndrome." *Pharmacogenomics*. 2007 Jan; 8(1):67-74.

Veale D, Kavanagh G, Fielding JF, Fitzgerald O. "Primary fibromyalgia and the irritable bowel syndrome: different expressions of a common pathogenetic process." *Br J Rheumatol*. 1991;30(3):220-222.

Cannon TD, Keller MC. "Endophenotypes in the genetic analysis of mental disorder." *Annu Rev Clin Psychol*. 2006; 2:267-290.

Korte SM, Koolhaas JM, Wingfield JC, McEwen BS. "The Darwinian concept of stress: benefits of allostasis and costs of allostatic load and the trade-offs in health and disease." *Neurosci Biobehav Rev*. 2005 Feb; 29(1):3-

38. Epub 2004 Dec 10.

Kroenke K, Spitzer RL. "Gender differences in the reporting of physical and somatoform symptoms." *Psychosom Med.* 1998; 60:150-155.

Gray J. *Men Are from Mars, Women Are from Venus: The Classic Guide to Understanding the Opposite Sex.* New York: Harper Paperbacks, 2004.

Kabat GC. *Hyping Health Risks: Environmental Hazards in Daily Life and the Science of Epidemiology.* New York: Columbia University Press, 2008.

Justice Felix Frankfurter, dissenting, *Henslee v. Union Planters Bank*, 335 U.S. 600 (1948).

Furmark T, Appel L, Henningsson S, Ahs F, Faria V, Linnman C, Pissiota A, Frans O, Bani M, Bettica P, Pich EM, Jacobsson E, Wahlstedt K, Oreland L, Långström B, Eriksson E, Fredrikson M. "A link between serotonin-related gene polymorphisms, amygdala activity, and placebo-induced relief from social anxiety." *J Neurosci.* 2008 Dec 3; 28(49):13066-74.

Chapter 12
YOUR Health and the Inner Life Tie That Binds

Moore T. *Care of the Soul: A Guide for Cultivating Depth and Sacredness in Everyday Life.* New York: HarperCollins Publishers, 1992.

Einstein A. as quoted in "What Life Means to Einstein," *The Saturday Evening Post*, vol. 202, October 26, 1929.

Buechner F. *Whistling in the Dark: An ABC Theologized.* New York: HarperCollins, 1988.

PART 3
THE IMBALANCED SELF

Chapter 13
We Are All Symptomatic: A New Model of Disease

Dacher E. *Intentional Healing: A Guide to the Mind-Body Healing System.* New York: Marlowe & Co, 1996.

Morris LB. "MIND AND BODY; She Feels Sick. The Doctor Can't Find Anything Wrong." *The New York Times*, June 24, 2001.

Fink P, Rosendal M. "Recent developments in the understanding and management of functional somatic symptoms in primary care." *Curr Opin*

Psychiatry. 2008; 21(2):182-8.

Dobson R. "Doctors rank myocardial infarction as most 'prestigious' disease and fibromyalgia as least." *BMJ.* 2007; 335:632.

Martinez-Lavin M. "Fibromyalgia conundrum: is scientific holism the answer?" *The Rheumatologist.* 2008;(2):26-27.

Frazier I. "Researchers Say." *The New Yorker.* December 9, 2002.

Gleick J. *Faster: The Acceleration of Just About Everything.* New York: Pantheon, 1999.

Friedman M, Rosenman R. *Type A Behavior and Your Heart.* New York: Knopf, 1974.

Thoreau HD. *Walden.* Boston: Ticknor and Fields, 1854.

Benson-Henry Institute for Mind Body Medicine. Available at: www.massgeneral.org/bhi/. Accessed 2 April, 2011.

McEwen BS. *The End of Stress As We Know It.* Washington, D. C.: National Academies Press, 2002.

Sapolsky R. *Why Zebras Don't Get Ulcers: The Acclaimed Guide to Stress, Stress-Related Diseases, and Coping (Third Edition).* New York: Henry Holt & Company, 2004.

Martinez-Lavin M, Vargas A. "Complex adaptive systems allostasis in fibromyalgia." *Rheum Dis Clin North Am.* 2009; 35(2):285-98.

Levine JA. *Move a Little, Lose a Lot.* New York: Crown, 2009.

Menninger K, Mayman M, Pruyser P. *The Vital Balance: The Life Process in Mental Health and Illness.* New York: Viking, 1963.

Meador CK. "The Last Well Person." *N Engl J Med.* 1994; 330:440-1.

Hadler NM. *Worried Sick: A Prescription for Health in an Overtreated America.* Chapel Hill, NC: The University of North Carolina Press, 2008.

Martinez-Lavin M, Infante O, Lerma C. "Hypothesis: the chaos and complexity theory may help our understanding of fibromyalgia and similar maladies." *Semin Arthritis Rheum.* 2008 Feb; 37(4):260-4. Epub 2007 June 14.

Sagan C, Druyan A. *The Demon-Haunted World: Science as a Candle in the Dark.* New York: Random House, 1996.

Chapter 14
How YOU Are Symptomatic: BODY TALK

Tolstoy LN. "Christianity and Patriotism." *The Kingdom of God and Peace: Essays.* London: Oxford University Press 1935.

Hassett AL, Clauw DJ. "Fibromyalgia and irritable bowel syndrome: is there a connection?" MedscapeCME Rheumatology. June 28, 2010.

Craig AD. "How do you feel — now? The anterior insula and human awareness." *Nat Rev Neurosci.* 2009 Jan; 10(1):59-70.

Blakeslee S, Blakeslee M. *The Body Has a Mind of Its Own: How Body Maps in Your Brain Help You Do (Almost) Everything Better.* New York: Random House, 2007.

Blakeslee S. "A Small Part of the Brain, and its Profound Effects." *The New York Times.* February 6, 2007.

Damasio A. *Descartes' Error: Emotion, Reason, and the Human Brain.* New York: Penguin Group, 2005.

Damasio A. *The Feeling of What Happens: Body and Emotion in the Making of Consciousness.* New York: Houghton Mifflin Harcourt, 2000.

Damasio A. *Looking for Spinoza: Joy, Sorrow, and the Feeling Brain.* New York: Houghton Mifflin Harcourt, 2003.

Martinez-Lavin M, Solano C. "Dorsal root ganglia, sodium channels, and fibromyalgia sympathetic pain." *Med Hypotheses* 2009; 72(1):64–6.

Martinez-Lavin M, Vargas A. "Complex adaptive systems allostasis in fibromyalgia." *Rheum Dis Clin North Am.* 2009 May; 35(2):285-98.

Williams DA, Clauw DJ. "Understanding fibromyalgia: lessons from the broader pain research community." J Pain. 2009; 10:777-791.

Ablin K, Clauw DJ. "From fibrositis to functional somatic syndromes to a bell-shaped curve of pain and sensory sensitivity: evolution of a clinical construct." Rheum Dis Clin North Am. 2009; 35:233-251.

Yunus MB. "Central sensitivity syndromes: a new paradigm and group nosology for fibromyalgia and overlapping conditions, and the related issue of disease versus illness." Semin Arthritis Rheum. 2008; 37:339-352.

The Rockefeller University. Featured Events: "Stress in the City." Public Lecture January 29, 2002. Available at: http://www.rockefeller.edu/lectures/stress012902.html. Accessed 2 April, 2011.

Chapter 15
Why YOU Are Symptomatic: STRESS RESPONSE

McEwen BS. *The End of Stress As We Know It.* Washington, D. C.: National Academies Press, 2002.

Kelly W. *The Pogo Papers.* New York: Simon & Schuster, 1953.

Benson-Henry Institute for Mind Body Medicine. Available at: http://www.massgeneral.org/bhi/. Accessed 2 April, 2011.

Gibran K. *The Prophet.* New York: Knopf Publishing Group, 1923.

Wang J, Rao H, Wetmore GS, Furlan PM, Korczykowski M, Dinges DF, Detre JA. "Perfusion functional MRI reveals cerebral blood flow pattern under psychological stress." *Proc Natl Acad Sci* U S A. 2005 Dec 6; 102(49):17804-9. Epub 2005 Nov 23.

Goode E. "The Heavy Cost of Chronic Stress." *The New York Times.* December 17, 2002.

Sapolsky R. *Why Zebras Don't Get Ulcers: The Acclaimed Guide to Stress, Stress-Related Diseases, and Coping (Third Edition).* New York: Henry Holt & Company, 2004.

McEwen BS. "Protective and damaging effects of stress mediators." *N Engl J Med.* 1998; 338: 171-179.

Mathieu P, Poirier P, Pibarot P, Lemieux I, Després JP. "Visceral obesity: the link among inflammation, hypertension, and cardiovascular disease." *Hypertension.* 2009 Apr; 53(4):577-84. Epub 2009 Feb 23.

Pashkow FJ, Libov C. *The Women's Heart Book: The Complete Guide to Keeping Your Heart Healthy* (Revised and Updated). New York: Hyperion, 2001.

Ablin K, Clauw DJ. "From fibrositis to functional somatic syndromes to a bell-shaped curve of pain and sensory sensitivity: evolution of a clinical construct." Rheum Dis Clin North Am. 2009; 35:233-251.

Chapter 16
Why YOU Are Symptomatic: EMOTION

McWhinney IR, Epstein RM, Freeman TR. "Lingua medica: rethinking somatization." *Annals Intern Med.* 1997 May 1; 126(9):747-50

National Institute of Mental Health. Available at: http://www.nimh.nih.gov/index.shtml. Accessed 2 April, 2011.

LeDoux J. The *Emotional Brain: The Mysterious Underpinnings of Emotional Life.* New York: Simon & Schuster, 1998.

Ekman P. *Emotions Revealed, Second Edition: Recognizing Faces and Feelings to Improve Communication and Emotional Life.* New York: Henry Holt & Company, 2007.

Pease B, Pease A. *The Definitive Book of Body Language: Why What People Say is Very Different from What They Think or Feel.* New York: Bantam Books, 2006.

DeSteno D. *Out of Character.* New York: Broadway Books, 2011 (in press).

DeSteno D. Social Emotions Group, Northeastern University. Available at: http://www.socialemotions.org/. Accessed 2 April, 2011.

Cannon WB. "Voices from the past. 'Voodoo' death." *Am J Public Health* 2002; 92:1593-6. (Original reference is: Cannon WB. "'Voodoo' death." *Am Anthropol* 1942; 44:169-81.)

MacLean P. "Psychosomatic disease and the 'visceral brain': recent developments bearing on the Papez theory of emotion." *Psychosom Med.* 1949; 11:338-53.

Chapter 17
Why YOU Are Symptomatic: CONSCIOUSNESS

Damasio A. *The Feeling of What Happens: Body and Emotion in the Making of Consciousness.* New York: Houghton Mifflin Harcourt, 2000.

Jung C. *Contributions to Analytical Psychology.* New York: Harcourt, Brace, and Company, 1928.

Merriam-Webster Online. Available at: http://www.merriam-webster.com/. Accessed 2 April, 2011.

"Mind & Body Special Issue. The Brain. A User's Guide." *Time.* January 29, 2007.

Winfrey O. Available at: www.oprah.com. Accessed 2 April, 2011.

Tolle E. *The Power of Now: A Guide to Spiritual Enlightenment.* Novato, California: New World Library, 2004.

Tolle E. *A New Earth: Awakening to Your Life's Purpose.* New York: Penguin Group, 2008.

Gibran K. *The Prophet.* New York: Knopf Publishing Group, 1923.

McEwen BS. *The End of Stress As We Know It.* Washington, D.C.: National Academies Press 2002.

Blakeslee S, Blakeslee M. *The Body Has a Mind of Its Own: How Body Maps in Your Brain Help You Do (Almost) Everything Better.* New York: Random House 2007.

Chapter 18
Why YOU May Be Symptomatic: SOUL

Steinbeck J. *Travels with Charley: In Search of America*. New York: Viking Press, 1962.

Dietrich B. as quoted in article by G. Jeffrey MacDonald, "Spiritual growth nurtured within." *USA TODAY*. January 14, 2008.

Goldstein NE. *God at the Edge: Searching for the Divine in Uncomfortable and Unexpected Places*. New York: Bell Tower, 2000.

Ephesians 4:26. *New American Standard Bible*. La Habra, California: The Lockman Foundation, 1995.

Lewis CS. *The Last Battle (The Chronicles of Narnia, Series #7)*.

Keck LR. *Healing as a Sacred Path*. West Chester, Pennsylvania: Swedenborg Foundation Publishers, 2002.

PART 4
REGAIN BALANCE
FIND HEALTH

YOU

Einstein A. as quoted in *Life* Magazine. May 2, 1955.

Rutecki GW. "A new spin on Malthus? Bad habits and prosperity are killing us." *Consultant*.2008; 48(8):571.

McNeil DG Jr. "Noninfectious illnesses are expected to become top killers within 20 years." *The New York Times*. June 3, 2008.

World Health Organization. "World Health Statistics 2008." Available at: www.who.int/whosis/whostat/2008/en/index.html. Accessed 2 April, 2011.

Reeves MJ, Rafferty AP. "Healthy lifestyle characteristics among adults in the United States, 2000." *Arch Intern Med*. 2005; 165:854-857.

Ford ES, Bergmann MM, Kroger J, Schienkiewilz A, Weikert C, Boeing H. "Healthy living is the best revenge: findings from the Euro Prospective Investigation into Cancer and Nutrition- Potsdam Study." *Arch Internal Med*. 2009 Aug. 10; 169(15) 1355-62.

Nagourney E. "Exercise: Working out the memory as well as the muscles." *The New York Times*, March 20, 2007.

Pereira AC, Huddleston DE, Brickman AM, Sosunov AA, Hen R, McKhann GM, Sloan R, Gage FH, Brown TR, Small SA. "An in vivo correlate of exercise-induced neurogenesis in the adult dentate gyrus." *Proc Natl Acad Sci U S A.* 2007 Mar 27; 104(13):5638-43. Epub 2007 Mar 20.

Carmichael M. "Stronger, Faster, Smarter." *Newsweek.* March 26, 2007.

Ratey JJ. *Spark: The Revolutionary New Science of Exercise and the Brain.* New York: Little, Brown and Company, 2008.

Eippert F, Finsterbusch J, Bingel U, Büchel C. "Direct evidence for spinal cord involvement in placebo analgesia." *Science.* 2009 Oct 16; 326(5951):404.

Brody H. *The Placebo Response: How You Can Release the Body's Inner Pharmacy for Better Health.* New York: HarperCollins Publishers, 2000.

Benson H. *Timeless Healing: The Power and Biology of Belief.* New York: Scribner, 1996.

Cannon WB. "Voices from the past. 'Voodoo' death." *Am J Public Health* 2002; 92:1593-6. (Original reference is: Cannon WB. "'Voodoo' death." *Am Anthropol* 1942; 44:169-81.)

Zautra AJ, Fasman R, Davis MC, Craig AD. "The effects of slow breathing on affective responses to pain stimuli: an experimental study." JPain. 2010 Apr; 149(1):12-8. Epub 2010 Jan 15.

Weil A. *8 Weeks to Optimum Health Revised Edition: A Proven Program for Taking Full Advantage of Your Body's Natural Healing Power.* New York: Knopf, 2006.

Massachusetts General Hospital Benson-Henry Institute for Mind Body Medicine. Available at: http://www.massgeneral.org/bhi/. Accessed 2 April, 2011.

"Eliciting the relaxation response." Available at: http://www.massgeneral.org/bhi/basics/eliciting_rr.aspx. Accessed 2 April, 2011.

FIND

Find YOUR Muse, Mentor, and Guide

Amen DG. *Change Your Brain, Change Your Body: Use Your Brain to Get and Keep the Body You Have Always Wanted.* New York: Harmony, 2010.

Imagine YOUR Own Wellness: Be Open, Unlearn, Rediscover

Einstein A. "What Life Means to Einstein." *The Saturday Evening Post,* vol. 202 October 26, 1929.

Nurture YOURSELF

Dine Well

National Heart Lung and Blood Institute: Obesity Education Initiative. "Calculate Your Body Mass Index." Available at: http://www.nhlbisupport.com/bmi/. Accessed 2 April, 2011.

American Heart Association. Available at: http://www.heart.org/HEARTORG/. Accessed 2 April, 2011.

American Heart Association. "My Fats Translator." Available at: http://www.heart.org/HEARTORG/GettingHealthy/FatsAndOils/Fats-Oils_UCM_001084_SubHomePage.jsp. Accessed 2 April, 2011.

Feinglos MN, Totten SE. "Are you what you eat, or how much you eat?" *Arch Intern Med.* 2008; 168(14):1485-1486.

Pollan M. *In Defense of Food: An Eater's Manifesto.* New York: Penguin Group, 2008.

Pollan M. Available at: www.michaelpollan.com. Accessed 2 April, 2011.

The Center for Mindful Eating. Available at: www.tcme.org. Accessed 2 April, 2011.

Duke Integrative Medicine. Available at: http://www.dukeintegrativemedicine.org/. Accessed 2 April, 2011.

Beck M. "Health Journal: Putting an End to Mindless Munching." *The Wall Street Journal.* May 13, 2008.

Hu FB. "Diet and cardiovascular disease prevention: the need for a paradigm shift" [editorial]. *J Am Coll Cardiol.* 2007 50(1):22-24. Epub 2007 June 18.

Pollan M. "Unhappy Meals." *The New York Times Magazine.* January 28, 2007.

Centers for Disease Control and Prevention. "Eat a Variety of Fruits and Vegetables Every Day." Available at: http://www.fruitsandveggiesmatter.gov/. Accessed 2 April, 2011.

Ornish D. *The Spectrum: A Scientifically Proven Program to Feel Better, Live Longer, Lose Weight, and Gain Health.* New York: Ballantine Books, 2007.

United States Department of Agriculture (USDA) Food Guide Pyramid. Available at: www.mypyramid.gov. Accessed 2 April, 2011.

Katzen M, Willett W. *Eat, Drink, and Weigh Less.* New York: Hyperion, 2006.

Harvard School of Public Health's Healthy Eating Pyramid. http://www.hsph.harvard.edu/nutritionsource/what-should-you-eat/pyramid/index.html. Accessed 2 April, 2011.

Agatston A. *The South Beach Diet.* New York: Rodale, 2003.

Agatston A. Available at: www.southbeachdiet.com. Accessed 2 April, 2011.

Weil A. Available at: www.drweil.com. Accessed 2 April, 2011.

Dr. Weil's Anti-Inflammatory Diet & Pyramid. Available at: http://www.drweil.com/drw/u/PAG00361/anti-inflammatory-food-pyramid.html. Accessed 2 April, 2011.

HEALTH

Hold YOUR Weight Down and Watch Your Waist

Pesmen C. "What Is Syndrome X?" *Best Life*, March, 2007.

Agatston A. *The South Beach Heart Health Revolution: Cardiac Prevention That Can Reverse Heart Disease and Stop Heart Attacks and Strokes (The South Beach Diet).* New York: St. Martin's Press, 2008 (first published as *The South Beach Heart Program.* New York: Rodale, 2006.)

Lopez-Jimenez F. Mayo *Clin Womens Healthsource.* 2008 Sep; 12(9):6.

Lee CD, Sui X, Blair SN. "Combined effects of cardiorespiratory fitness, not smoking, and normal waist girth on morbidity and mortality in men." *Arch Intern Med.* 2009 Dec 14; 169(22):2096-101.

Exercise Regularly

Rowe JW, Kahn RL. *Successful Aging.* New York: Dell, 1999.

Department of Health and Human Services; US Department of Agriculture. "Dietary guidelines for Americans." Available at: http://health.gov/dietaryguidelines/. Accessed 2 April, 2011.

"Physical Activity and Public Health Updated Recommendations for Adults" from the American College of Sports Medicine and the American Heart Association (ACSM/AHA Recommendations). Available at: http://www.heart.org/HEARTORG/GettingHealthy/PhysicalActivity/GettingActive/Getting-Active_UCM_001189_SubHomePage.jsp. Accessed 2 April, 2011.

Agatston A. *The South Beach Heart Health Revolution: Cardiac Prevention That Can Reverse Heart Disease and Stop Heart Attacks and Strokes (The South Beach Diet).* New York: St. Martin's Press, 2008 (first published as *The South Beach Heart Program.* New York: Rodale, 2006.)

"Shape Up America: Physical Activity Calculator." Available at: http://www.shapeup.org/interactive/phys1.php. Accessed 2 April, 2011.

Add Vitamins/Supplements

Weil A. *Healthy Aging: A Lifelong Guide to Your Physical and Spiritual Well-Being.* New York: Alfred A. Knopf, 2005.

Weil A. Available at: www.drweil.com. Accessed 2 April, 2011.

Christen WG, Glynn RJ, Chew EY, Albert CM, Manson, JE. "Folic acid, pyridoxine, and cyanocobalamin combination treatment and age-related macular degeneration in women: the women's antioxidant and folic acid cardiovascular study." *Arch Intern Med.* 2009; 169(4):335-341.

Autier P, Gandini S. "Vitamin D supplementation and total mortality." *Arch Intern Med* 2007; 167(16):1730-1737.

Holick M. "Vitamin D deficiency." *N Engl J Med* 2007; 357:266-81.

"Plant stanol/sterol esters and risk of coronary artery disease." US Food and Drug Administration, Center for Food Safety and Applied Nutrition. A Food Labeling Guide – Appendix C. September 1994 (Editorial revisions June 1999 and November, 2000).

Sommerfeld, J. "Dietary supplements face stricter regulations: for first time, companies must test products for contamination, FDA says." MSNBC. Available at: http://www.msnbc.msn.com/id/19370824/. Accessed 2 April, 2011.

Finn R. "Consumer probiotics may make too many health claims." *Internal Medicine News.* July 15, 2008.

Learn How Doctors Think and How to Work with Them

Groopman J. *How Doctors Think.* New York: Houghton Mifflin, 2007.

Healy B. "Medicine, the Art." *U.S. News & World Report.* July 14, 2007.

Goldstein J. "As Doctors Get a Life, Strains Show. Quest for Free Time Reshapes Medicine; A 'Team' Approach." *The Wall Street Journal.* April 29, 2008.

Conrad P. *The Medicalization of Society: On the Transformation of Human Conditions into Treatable Disorders.* Baltimore: The Johns Hopkins University Press, 2007.

Parker-Pope T. "Well; Doctor and Patient, Now at Odds." *The New York Times,* July 29, 2008.

Jauhar S. *Intern: A Doctor's Initiation.* New York: Farrar, Straus and Giroux, 2009.

Jauhar S. "The Instincts to Trust Are Usually the Patient's." *The New York Times.* January 6, 2009.

Smith RC. *Patient-Centered Interviewing: An Evidence-Based Method.* Philadelphia: Lippincott Williams and Wilkins, 2002.

Smith RC, Lyles JS, Gardiner JC, Sirbu C, Hodges A, Collins C, Dwamena FC, Lein C, William Given C, Given B, Goddeeris J. "Primary care clinicians treat patients with medically unexplained symptoms: a randomized controlled trial." *J Gen Intern Med.* 2006 Jul; 21(7):671-7.

Jackson JL, O'Malley PG, Kroenke K. "Clinical predictors of mental disorders among medical outpatients: validation of the 'S4' model." *Psychosomatics.* 1998; 39:431–6.

Kroenke K, Spitzer RL, Williams JBW, Monahan PO, Löwe B. "Anxiety disorders in primary care: prevalence, impairment, comorbidity, and detection." *Ann Intern Med.* 2007; 146:317-325.

Kroenke K, Spitzer RL, Williams JB. "The Patient Health Questionnaire-2: validity of a two-item depression screener." *Med Care.* 2003 Nov; 41(11):1284-92.

Agency for Healthcare Research and Quality (AHRQ). "Patient Health Questionnaire (PHQ2)." Available at: http://innovations.ahrq.gov/content. aspx?id=2280. Accessed 2 April, 2011.

Agatston A. *The South Beach Heart Health Revolution: Cardiac Prevention That Can Reverse Heart Disease and Stop Heart Attacks and Strokes (The South Beach Diet).* New York: St. Martin's Press, 2008 (first published as *The South Beach Heart Program.* New York: Rodale, 2006.)

Blaha MJ, Bansal S, Rouf R, Golden SH, Blumenthal RS, Defilippis AP. "A practical 'ABCDE' approach to the metabolic syndrome." *Mayo Clin Proc.* 2008 Aug; 83(8):932-41.

HealthVault (Microsoft®). Available at: http://www.healthvault.com. Accessed 2 April, 2011.

Google Health (Google™). Available at: www.google.com/health. Accessed 2 April, 2011.

United States Department of Health & Human Services Surgeon General's Family History Initiative. Available at: http://www.hhs.gov/ familyhistory/. Accessed 2 April, 2011.

The UNC Center for Functional GI & Motility Disorders. Dalton CB,

Drossman DA. The Use of Antidepressants in the Treatment of Irritable Bowel Syndrome and Other Functional GI Disorders. Available at: http://www.med.unc.edu/ibs. Patient Education/Educational GI Handouts/Irritable Bowel Syndrome (IBS)/IBS and Antidepressants. Accessed 2 April, 2011.

Jackson JL, O'Malley PG, Kroenke K. "Antidepressants and cognitive-behavioral therapy for symptom syndromes." *CNS Spectr.* 2006 Mar; 11(3):212-22.

Team with All Care-Givers

Pruyser P. *The Minister as Diagnostician: Personal Problems in Pastoral Perspective.* Philadelphia: Westminster John Knox Press, 1976.

Mustapha IZ, Debrey S, Oladubu M, Ugarte R. "Markers of systemic bacterial exposure in periodontal disease and cardiovascular disease risk: a systematic review and meta-analysis." *JPeriodontol.* 2007 Dec; 78(12):2289-302.

Help Others Help Themselves

Olde Hartman T, Hassink-Franke L, Dowrick C, Fortes S, Lam C, van der Horst H, Lucassen P, van Weel-Baumgarten E. "Medically unexplained symptoms in family medicine: defining a research agenda." Proceedings from WONCA 2007. *Fam Pract.* 2008 Aug; 25(4):266-71. Epub 2008 Jul 1.

INDEX

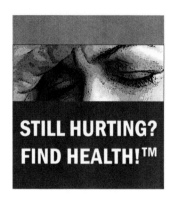

We Want to Hear From YOU!

JOIN THE Still Hurting? FIND HEALTH!™ Community

Everyone hurts.

This book is the first of the Still Hurting? FIND HEALTH ™ series.

Become a member of the Still Hurting? FIND HEALTH! ™ community on the website, so that you can remain updated and we all learn from one another. Join the mailing list. After you have read the book, post your review and comments on the website and online where you purchased it.

A reading guide is available on the website at:

stillhurtingfindhealth.com/Book-Club-Reading-Guide.html

stillhurtingfindhealth.com

3/12 Withdrawn.

For Every
Individual...

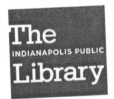

Renew by Phone
269-5222

Renew on the Web
www.imcpl.org

For General Library Infomation
please call 275-4100

CPSIA information can be obtained at www.ICGtesting.com
Printed in the USA
241022LV00002B/156/P